OXFORD MEDICAL PUBLICATIONS

Interventional
Radiology

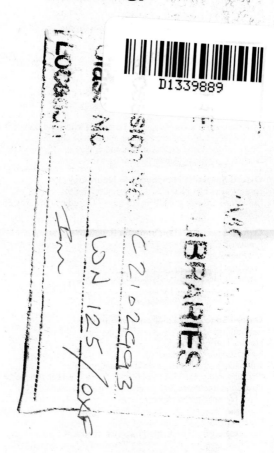

Published and forthcoming Oxford Specialist Handbooks

General Oxford Specialist Handbooks
A Resuscitation Room Guide (Banerjee and Hargreaves)

Oxford Specialist Handbooks in End of Life Care
Cardiology: From advanced disease to bereavement (Beattie, Connelly, and Watson eds.)
Nephrology: From advanced disease to bereavement (Brown, Chambers, and Eggeling)

Oxford Specialist Handbooks in Anaesthesia
Cardiac Anaesthesia (Barnard and Martin eds.)
Neuroanaesthesia (Nathanson and Moppett eds.)
Obstetric Anaesthesia (Clyburn, Collis, Harries, and Davies eds.)
Paediatric Anaesthesia (Doyle ed.)

Oxford Specialist Handbooks in Cardiology
Cardiac Catheterization and Coronary Angiography (Mitchell, West, Leeson, and Banning)
Pacemakers and ICDs (Timperley, Leeson, Mitchell, and Betts eds.)
Echocardiography (Leeson, Mitchell, and Becher eds.)
Heart Failure (Gardner, McDonagh, and Walker)
Nuclear Cardiology (Sabharwal, Loong, and Kelion)

Oxford Specialist Handbooks in Neurology
Epilepsy (Alarcon, Nashef, Cross, and Nightingale)
Parkinson's Disease and Other Movement Disorders (Edwards, Bhatia, and Quinn)

Oxford Specialist Handbooks in Paediatrics
Paediatric Gastroenterology, Hepatology, and Nutrition (Beattie, Dhawan, and Puntis eds.)
Paediatric Nephrology (Rees, Webb, and Brogan)
Paediatric Neurology (Forsyth and Newton eds.)
Paediatric Oncology and Haematology (Bailey and Skinner eds.)
Paediatric Radiology (Johnson, Williams, and Foster)

Oxford Specialist Handbooks in Surgery
Cardiothoracic Surgery (Chikwe, Beddow, and Glenville)
Hand Surgery (Warwick)
Neurosurgery (Samandouras)
Operative Surgery (McLatchie and Leaper eds.)
Otolaryngology and Head and Neck Surgery (Warner and Corbridge)
Plastic and Reconstructive Surgery (Giele and Cassell eds.)
Renal Transplantation (Talbot)
Urological Surgery (Reynard, Sullivan, Turner, Feneley, Armenakas, and Mark eds.)
Vascular Surgery (Hands, Murphy, Sharp, and Ray-Chaudhuri eds.)

Oxford Specialist Handbooks in Radiology

Interventional Radiology

Dr Raman Uberoi

Consultant Interventional Radiologist,
John Radcliffe Hospital,
Oxford, UK.

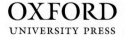

OXFORD
UNIVERSITY PRESS

OXFORD
UNIVERSITY PRESS

Great Clarendon Street, Oxford OX2 6DP

Oxford University Press is a department of the University of Oxford.
It furthers the University's objective of excellence in research, scholarship,
and education by publishing worldwide in

Oxford New York

Auckland Cape Town Dar es Salaam Hong Kong Karachi
Kuala Lumpur Madrid Melbourne Mexico City Nairobi
New Delhi Shanghai Taipei Toronto

With offices in

Argentina Austria Brazil Chile Czech Republic France Greece
Guatemala Hungary Italy Japan Poland Portugal Singapore
South Korea Switzerland Thailand Turkey Ukraine Vietnam

Oxford is a registered trade mark of Oxford University Press
in the UK and in certain other countries

Published in the United States
by Oxford University Press Inc., New York

© Oxford University Press, 2009

The moral rights of the author have been asserted
Database right Oxford University Press (maker)

First published 2009

British Library Cataloguing in Publication Data
Data available

Library of Congress Cataloging in Publication Data
Data available

Typeset by Cepha Imaging Private Ltd., Bangalore, India
Printed in Italy
on acid-free paper by
L.E.G.O. S.p.A.

ISBN 978–0–19–954772–2

10 9 8 7 6 5 4 3 2 1

To my parents Radhesham and Vimla Uberoi.
My wife Susan and my boys Jamie and Adam
for being so patient and understanding.

Contents

Detailed contents

Acknowledgements

I am grateful to the following companies for their assistance in providing high quality images for this book.

Abbot Vascular, Maidenhead, UK
Amplatzer Medical UK LTD
Arrow International UK LTD, Uxbridge, UK
Bard, Crawley, West Sussex, UK
Boston Scientific, St Albans, Herts, UK
BVM Medical, BVM House, Hinkley UK
Cooks (UK) LTD Letchworth, Garden City, Hertfordshire UK.
Cordis Endovascular South Ascot, Berkshire UK
EV3 LTD Bishops Stortford, Herts UK
Lombard Medical, Didcot, Oxfordshire, UK
Pyramed LTD, Salisbury, Wiltshire, UK
St Jude
Terumo UK LTD, Egham, Surrey UK

List of Abbreviations

AP	antero-posterior
APPT	activated partial throboplastin time
AT	anterior tibial artery
ATM	atomospheres
AVM	arteriovenous malformation
BP	blood pressure
BMC	biliary manipulation catheter
CFA	common femoral artery
CFV	common femoral vein
CIA	common iliac artery
CIN	contrast induced nephropathy
CPP	chronic pelvic pain
CT	computed tomography
CVC	central venous catheter
CXR	chest xray
DSA	digital subtraction angiography
DVT	deep vein thrombosis
ECG	electrocardiogram
ECST	European Carotid Surgery Trial
EIA	external iliac artery
EUS	endoscopic ultrasonography
EVAR	endovascular aortic aneurysm repair
F	French i.e 1F=0.33mm
FB	foreign body
FMH	Fibromuscular hyperplasia
FNAC	fine needle aspiration cytology
G	gauge
GI	gastro-intestinal
GOJ	gastro-oesophogel junction
HDU	high dependency unit
ICA	internal carotid artery
IJV	internal jugular vein
INR	international normalised ratio
IM	intramuscular
IMA	inferior mesenteric artery
IV	intravenous

IVC	inferior vena cava
LA	local anaesthetic
LAO	left anterior oblique
µg	micrograms
Mg	milligram
Ml	mililiters
MR	magnetic resonance
NASCET	North American Symptomatic Carotid Endarterectomy
NG	nasogastric
O	oral
PCS	pelvic congestion syndrome
PEG	percutaneous enteral gastrostomy
PE	pulmonary embolus
PIG	percutaneously inserted gastrostomy
PT	posterior tibial artery
PTA	percutaneous transluminal angioplasty
PVA	plyvinal alchohol
PVD	peripheral vascular disease
RAO	right anterior oblique
RF	radiofrequency
RIG	radiologicaly inserted gastrostomy
rTPA	tissue plasminogen activater
SC	subcutaneous
SCVIR	Society of Cardiovascular and Interventional Radiology
SMA	superior mesenteric artery
SL	sublingual
STD	sodium tetraethyl deconeoate
SVCO	superior vena cava obstruction
TASC	transatlantic consensus
TAE	transcatheter arterial embolization
TAE	therapeutic arterial embolization
TACE	transcatheter arterial chemo-embolization
TACE	chemoembolization
TPA	tissue plasminogen activater
UAE	uterine artery embolization
US/USG	ultrasonography

List of drugs

Abciximab
Acetaminophen
Acetylcysteine
Amethocaine hydrochloride
Amlodipine
Ampicillin
Aquinolone
Atropine
Augementin®
Barium sulphate
Bendroflumethiazide
Benzodiazepines
Beraprost
Bisoprolol
Bivalirudin
Bosentan
Bupivacaine
Bupropion
Buscopan®
Brevibloc®
Captopril
Catapres®
Cephalosporin
Chlorhexidine
Cilostazol
Cimetidine
Cinnarizine
Ciprofloxacin
Cisplatin
Clonidine
Clopidogrel
Cilostazol
Dalteparin
Definity®
Dextran 40
Diazepam
Diclofenac
Diphenhydramine
Doxorubicin
EMLA
Epinephrine
Esmolol
Fenoldapam
Fentanyl
Flumazenil
Furosemide

Heparin
Gadodiamide
Gadolinium
Gadopentate dimeglumine
Gadoterate meglumine
Gadoversetamide
Gentamicin
Gliclazide
Glitazones
Glubran
Glucagon
Glyceryl trinitrate
Glycopyrrolate
Heparin
Ibuprofen
Iloprost
Inositol nicotinate
Iodixanol
Iohexol
Iopamidol
Iopromide
Iotrol
Ioversol
Ioxaglate
Isovue®
Ketamine
Labetalol
Leucovorin
Lidocaine
Lipiodol
Lorazepam
Lopirin
Magnevist®
Metformin
Methyl-prednisolone
Metronidazole
Midazolam
Mitomycin
Morphine
Naftidrofuryl
Naloxone
Naproxen
Nifedipine
Nitroprusside
Omnipaque™
Omniscan™

Optimark®
Optiray™
Pentoxifylline
Pentoxigylline
Perflutren
Prednisolone
Propofol
Quinolone
Ramipril
Remifentanil
Reteplase
Rosiglitazone
Simvastatin
Sono Vue®
Streptokinase

Sufentanil
Sulphonylureas
Tenecteplase
TISSEEL®
Theophylline
Ticlopidine
TPA
Trandate
Ultravist®
Urokinase
Verapamil
Warfarin
Xylocaine

Contributors list

Suzie Anthony
Consultant Interventional
Radiologist,
Oxford Radcliffe Hospitals NHS
Trust, UK

Sriharsha Athreya
Assistant Professor,
McMaster University,
Angio Interventional Radiologist,
St. Joseph's Healthcare,
Hamilton, Canada

Philip Boardman
Consultant Radiologist,
Churchill Hospital, Headington,
Oxford, UK

Gareth Bydawell
Interventional Fellow,
St George's Hospital,
London, UK

Arul Ganeshan
Clinical Interventional Fellow,
University of British Columbia,
Vancouver, Canada

Michael Gonsalves
Specialist Registrar,
Department of St Radiology,
George's Hospital,
London, UK

Richard J. Hughes
Consultant Radiologist,
Buckinghamshire Hospitals NHS
Trust, UK

Atique Imam
Specialist Registrar, Department of
Radiology,
John Radcliffe Hospital,
Oxford, UK

Sumaira Macdonald
Consultant Vascular Radiologist &
Honorary Clinical Senior Lecturer,
Freeman Hospital,
Newcastle upon Tyne, UK

Navin B. Mathias
Consultant Interventional
Radiologist,
Hairmyres Hospital,
Glasgow, UK

Uday Patel
Consultant Radiologist,
St George's Hospital and
Medical School,
London, UK

Praveen Peddu
Consultant Radiologist (Special
interest: Hepatobiliary and inter-
vention),
King's College Hospital
London, UK

Jane Phillips-Hughes
Consultant Radiologist,
John Radcliffe Hospital,
Oxford, UK

Peter Rowlands
Consultant in Radiology,
Royal Liverpool University
Hospital, UK

Paul S. Sidhu
Consultant Radiologist and Senior
Lecturer,
King's College Hospital
London, UK

Dinuke R Warakaulle
Consultant Interventional
Radiologist,
Stoke Manderville Hospital,
Aylesbury, UK

Introduction

Interventional radiology is an exciting new subspecialty which has delivered major advances in the treatment of patients with minimally invasive techniques. It has promised much over the last two decades and delivered precision therapy replacing some well established surgical techniques as well as complimenting others, allowing treatment of patients in whom it would otherwise have been considered too dangerous.

It is vital for any aspiring interventionist to have a profound clinical knowledge in their area of interest as well as acquiring the fundamental catheter and guidewire skills which form the basis of the majority of intervention. Good training is vital to maintain high standards in the specialty. There is no substitute to being formally trained in a good interventional programme and gaining the bedrock of skills on which the young interventionist can then build upon. This book aims to give the reader a detailed guide on carrying out many of these procedures, including tricks and tips from highly experienced experts with many years of experience in the field of intervention. This book is designed to be a companion which can be carried around in the pocket and used to help the trainee and young interventionist when dealing with the simplest to the most complex of cases. It should be viewed as having a senior colleague on hand for advice and tips.

One of the important elements of intervention is becoming familiar with the key pieces of equipment and their use and this has been one of the major focuses in this book.

'You young beginning surgeons, open your ears and remember with diligence this short word. When you are called to a patient, if the matter appears to you too difficult or not entirely familiar do not be ashamed to send after one or two other surgeons so that they can help you and give you good advice from which you and the patient can derive great benefit...if everything goes well, you will share in the success. If things go wrong, they will share the burden.'

Hieronymous Brunschwig – from the Book of Cirurgia, 1497

Introduction

Informed consent

Informed consent

This section is designed to provide a brief overview of consent, for a more detailed explanation readers are advised to read the GMC guidance on this subject.

This can be complex and difficult and you should seek advice from the hospital administration or your medical defence union.

Who can take consent?

- Ideally this should be the doctor who is going to undertake the procedure but it can be any appropriately trained health professional who is familiar with the procedure and is aware of the risks and complications.

Provide sufficient information

- The details of the diagnosis and prognosis, and the likely prognosis if the condition is left untreated.
- The uncertainties about the diagnosis including the options for further investigation prior to treatment.
- The options for treatment or management of the condition, including the option not to treat.
- The purpose of a proposed investigation or treatment; details of the procedures or therapies involved, including subsidiary treatment such as methods of pain relief; how the patient should prepare for the procedure; and details of what the patient might experience during or after the procedure including common and serious side effects.
- For each option, explanations of the likely benefits and the probabilities of success; discussion of any serious or frequently occurring risks and of any lifestyle changes which may be caused by, or necessitated by, the treatment.
- Advice about whether a proposed treatment is experimental.
- How and when the patient's condition and any side effects will be monitored or re-assessed.
- The name of the doctor who will have overall responsibility for the treatment and, where appropriate, the names of the senior members of his or her team.
- Whether doctors in training will be involved, and the extent to which students may be involved in the investigation or treatment.
- A reminder that patients are entitled to change their minds about a decision at any time.
- A reminder that patients have a right to seek a second opinion.
- Where applicable, the details of any costs or charges which the patient may have to meet.
- You must respond honestly to any questions that the patient raises and, as far as possible, answer as fully as the patient wishes.
- Use up-to-date written material, visual and other aids to explain the complex aspects of the investigation, diagnosis or treatment.
- Wherever possible meet particular language and communication needs.
- Where appropriate, discuss with patients the possibility of bringing a relative or friend to the consultation, or of making a tape recording of the consultation.

- Explain the probabilities of success, or the risk of failure, or the harm associated with the options for treatment, using accurate data.
- Allow patients sufficient time to reflect, before and after making a decision, especially where the information is complex or the severity of the risks is great. Where patients have difficulty understanding information, or there is a lot of information to absorb, it may be appropriate to provide it in manageable amounts, with appropriate written or other back-up material, over a period of time, or to repeat it.
- Involve nursing or other members of the health care team in discussions with the patient, where appropriate.
- Ensure that, where treatment is not to start until some time after consent has been obtained, the patient is given a clear avenue for reviewing their decision with the person providing the treatment.

Ensuring voluntary decision making
- Give a balanced view of the options.
- Explain the need for informed consent.

Emergencies
In an emergency, where consent cannot be obtained, you may provide medical treatment to anyone who needs it, provided the treatment is limited to what is immediately necessary in order to save life or avoid a significant deterioration in the patient's health. However, you must still respect the terms of any valid advance refusal which you know about, or which are drawn to your attention. You should tell the patient what has been done, and why, as soon as the patient has recovered sufficiently to understand.

'Best interests' principle
In deciding what options may be reasonably considered as being in the best interests of a patient who lacks the capacity to decide, you should take into account:
- The options for treatment or investigation which are indicated clinically.
- Any evidence of the patient's previously expressed preferences, including an advance statement.
- Your own and the health care team's knowledge of the patient's background, such as any cultural, religious, or employment considerations.
- Any views about the patient's preferences stated by a third party who may have other knowledge of the patient, for example the patient's partner, family, carer, tutor-dative (Scotland), or a person with parental responsibility.
- Which option least restricts the patient's future choices, where more than one option (including non-treatment) seems reasonable in the patient's best interests.

Key points
- Patients, whether adult or child, need to know what is happening to them and why.
- What are the major or most frequently occurring complications and risks?

- What benefits are there in having the procedure and what are the risks in not having it?
- The probability of success and alternative options.
- Will the results be long lasting?
- What are the options if it fails or recurs?
- Ask if the patients have any questions.

It is always best practice, for common procedures, to have leaflets or literature available for patients prior to the procedure. Many of these are available online from the RCR or SCVIR websites and will enable patients to have the time to understand and have questions ready.

Always use language a lay person can understand and ideally consent out of the interventional suite and on the ward or pre-assessment clinic in a non threatening environment.

A discussion may also take place on the phone prior to admission in order to save time.

Check again, immediately prior to procedure if they wish to undergo the procedure or if there are any issues.

Further reading

General Medical Council. Seeking patients' consent: The ethical considerations. London GMC Publications, 178 Great Portland street, London W1N 6JE.

Chapter 2

Drugs, sedation, and analgesia

Introduction

Pharmaceutical agents including sedatives, anxiolytics, analgesics, antico-agulant, thrombolytic, antihypertensive, antilipid, and antiplatelets agents as well a variety of contrast agents are used in the day-to-day practice of interventional radiology. A brief description of the common drugs used routinely in interventional procedures is given below.

Medications pre-intervention

Managing risk factors before intervention

Smoking
- Most important aetiological risk factor for peripheral arterial disease (PAD).
- Smoking increases the risk for PAD by 4.23 times.
- Smoking increases the risk of amputation in persons with intermittent claudication.
- Patency in lower extremity bypass grafts is worse in smokers than in non smokers.
- Cessation of smoking decreases the progression of PAD to critical leg ischaemia and decreases the risk of myocardial infarction (MI) and death from vascular causes.
- Cessation of smoking is the most clinically efficacious and cost-effective intervention for the treatment of PAD.

Management: includes
- Use of nicotine patches or nicotine polacrilex gum.
- If this is unsuccessful, a nicotine nasal spray and/or treatment with the antidepressant bupropion should be considered.
- A nicotine inhaler is also available.

Hypertension (Systolic >130 mmHg and diastolic >80 mmHg)
- Established risk factor for PAD.
- Increases the risk of PAD by 1.75 times.
- Much of the evidence for treating hypertension with PAD extrapolated from data from coronary artery disease (CAD).

Management includes
- Lifestyle modifications.
- Drug therapy.

Indications for therapy
- Very high blood pressure values (>180/110Hg).
- Cardiovascular disease.
- Three or more cardiovascular risk factors (age: men >55 yrs, women >65 yrs, smoking, dyslipidemia, positive family history, obesity, CRP >1 mg/Dl.
- Endorgan disease (LVH, microalbuminuria, raised createnine).
- Diabetes mellitus.

There are many different regimes which are equally effective, i.e. diuretics, betablockers and newer agents such as calcium blockers and ACE inhibitors.

There is no evidence that β blockers adversely affect claudication.

- An ACE should be the first line of defence in the presence of congestive heart failure, diabetes mellitus with proteinuria and post MI with systolic left ventricular dysfunction, i.e. ramipril – commence with 1.25 mg/day increasing to a maximum of 10mg/day .
- A beta blocker should be prescribed following an acute MI, i.e. bisoprolol – 10 mg/day.
- A diuretic (bendroflumethiazide 2.5 mg/day) or long acting calcium blocker (amlodipine 5mg/day to max. of 10 mg/day) may be more effective in the elderly with isolated hypertension.

Diabetes
- Diabetes is a risk factor for PAD.
- Increases risk of PAD by 2.08 times.
- Diabetes should be treated so that the haemoglobin A_{1c} level decreases to <7% and the incidence of MI is consequently reduced.

In addition to the management of diet oral hypoglycaemics such as metformin (500mg/day increasing initially to 1500 mg to a maximum of 2 g), glitazones (rosiglitazone 4 mg–8 mg) and sulfonylureas (gliclazide 40–80 mg to a maximum of 160 mg) are typically used for type 2 diabetes.

Insulin may be required, in addition, if HgA1C remains >7% and for type 1 diabetes.

Dyslipidemia
- Hypercholesterolaemia increases the risk of PAD by 1.67 times –treatment with statins reduces the incidence of mortality, cardiovascular events and stroke in PAD with and without CAD.
- Simvastatin significantly reduces the incidence of intermittent claudication by 38% compared with a placebo.
- Statins also reduce atherosclerotic aneurysm degeneration of arteries.

Therefore all patients with PAD and hypercholesterolaemia should be treated with statins in order to reduce cardiovascular mortality and morbidity, reduce the progression of PAD and improve exercise time until intermittent claudication.

The aim is to maintain LDL <100 mg/dL and with those >40 years of age with overt cardiovascular disease a 30–40% reduction regardless of baseline (i.e. simvastatin – 10–80 mg single nightly dose).

Drug treatment of claudication
Five oral drugs have been licensed for the treatment of claudication. Two of these, inositol nicotinate and cinnarizine, have not been established as effective when compared with a placebo.

- Pentoxifylline (400 mg 3 times per day) improves walking distance by 29 metres over a placebo (50% compared with baseline in the placebo; pentoxigylline provides an additional 30% improvement).
- Naftidrofuryl has shown an increased walking distance of up to 30% compared to a placebo at 6 months.

- Cilostazol (100 mg orally 2 times a day), a phosphodiesterase inhibitor, shows a 40% increase in walking distance at 3 months and is the drug of choice in the management of claudication.

Ulcers
- Ticlopidine has also been shown to be effective and has also been effective in the healing of ulcers.
- Unfractionated heparin used as an prophylaxis and as an adjuvant treatment to vascular procedures. Low molecular weight heparin (LMWH) has also shown beneficial results in the healing of ischaemic ulcers.
- There is no additional benefit in using oral anti-coagulants.
- Prostaglandin analogues: IV PGI_2 & PGE or oral beraprost have an antiplatelet and vasodilator effect. Iloprost is shown to heal arterial ulcers. An intra-arterial bolus of 3000 ng is given followed by 2 ng/Kg/min/day up to 7 days.

Increased plasma homocysteine level is a risk factor for PAD, but there is no data to show any benefit in terms of reduction.

Management of pre-existing medications before intervention

Warfarin
If this can be discontinued it should be stopped at least 3 days prior to intervention and INR checked the day before. An INR of 1.5 or less is adequate.

If not, i.e mechanical valve, the patient will need to be admitted and commenced on heparin.

In an emergency fresh frozen plasma may be given and a closure device used.

Heparin
Stopping heparin 3 hours before intervention is usually adequate without the need to check APTT.

Aspirin
All patients should be commenced on lifelong aspirin 75–325 mg/day as soon as a diagnosis of peripheral vascular disease is made with no need to stop prior to procedure.

Clopidogrel
This is usually employed for coronary stents. It is not necessary to stop prior to the procedure but one should consider using a closure device.

Diabetic drugs
Metformin: stop for 48 hours post procedure and check renal functions before restarting.

Other oral hypoglycaemics: stop on the morning of the procedure and restart when taking food.

Insulin dependent: reduce the morning dose, i.e. by 50% with a 5% dextrose infusion with regular blood glucose measurements. A sliding scale is rarely needed.

Prescription of specific medications before intervention

Contrast induced nephropathy (CIN)

Defined as an elevation of serum creatine >25% or 44micromole/l within 3 days of contrast administration.

Risk factors for CIN

- Pre-existing RF.
- Age.
- Dehydration.
- Heart failure.
- Current use of NSAIDs.

Management

- Prehydration (100 mls/hr of saline. Start the infusion 4 hrs prior to the contrast administration and continue the infusion for next 24 hrs) and consider use of LOCM and bicarbonate to reduce the risk of CIN .
- N- acetyl cysteine (150 mg/Kg iv pre and 50 mg/Kg iv post) and ascorbic acid may be valuable in the case of a very high risk patient although the data are conflicting.

Antiplatelets

- Platelets and their products play a key role in arteriosclerosis.
- Platelet aggregability is 30% higher in patients with peripheral vascular disease even if asymptomatic.
- Claudication progression is reduced with antiplatelet-treatment.
- Anti-platelet therapy has also shown considerable reductions in fatal and non fatal vascular events in high-risk vascular patients.
- The risk reduction for antiplatelet therapy versus placebo is 46% for non fatal stroke, 32% for non fatal myocardial infarction, and 20% for death from a vascular cause.
- Even in low risk patients, antiplatelet therapy shows considerable risk reduction.
- Patients treated by peripheral angioplasty benefit from receiving aspirin at a dose of 50 mg to 300 mg daily, started prior to PTA and continued for at least 2 years or life-long.
- Thienopyridines, e.g. clopidogrel (75 mg /day), are a useful alternative where aspirin is not tolerated, there is aspirin resistance or as a combination therapy with aspirin where there are increased risk factors for re-occlusion. Clopidogrel (75 mg/day)shows a greater cardiovascular risk reduction compared to aspirin, but clopidogrel is more expensive.
- Abciximab (250 µg/kg iv over 1 minute then 125 nanograms/Kg/min to max. of 10 mcg/min) might also be a useful drug for extended femoro-popliteal interventions in patients with high risk for re-occlusion.

Unexpected uncontrolled hypertension

The SCVIR defines this as diastolic >100 mmHg and systolic pressure >180 mmHg. This can result in bleeding from the wound peri and post procedure.

Administer 10 mg oral nifedipine up to 30 mg at 20 minute intervals. It works quickest given sublingually, but it is vital to monitor the patient's ECG, pulse, and BP.

Medications during intervention

Local anesthetic drugs

- Lidocaine: A mid local anesthetic agent. Rapid onset (2–5 min). Median duration of action (60 mins). Commonly used at needle puncture sites prior to interventional procedures. Co-administration with epinephrine can increase duration up to 3 hrs. Avoid epinephrine in areas of limited blood supply (ears, noses) or in distal appendages (fingers, toes, penis) in order to reduce risk of local necrosis.
- Bupivacaine: A mid LA agent. Slow onset (5–10 mins) with a long duration (4 hrs) of action. Can be prolonged with epinephrine. A combination of lidocaine, bupivacaine and epinephrine can be used to produce a rapid onset with prolonged analgesic effect.
- EMLA: A eutectic mixture of lidocaine and prilocaine. A good LA applied to the skin 1 hour before needle puncture in the paediatric population.

Anti-coagulation

- Heparin: It is standard practice to give 3–5,000 units during the procedure in divided doses. This is increased for longer procedures, i.e. >2 hours. Ideally doses should be titrated with an activated clotting time of 250–300 seconds.
- Low molecular weight heparins (dalteparin sodium 2,500 units) might also be superior to unfractionated heparin to prevent early and mid-term re-occlusion/re-stenosis after femoro-popliteal angioplasty.
- Bivalirudin may be used as an alternative (750 mcg/Kg i.v. pre-procedure then 1.75 mg/Kg/hr for up to 4 hours).

Fibrinolytic drugs

- These drugs (e.g. streptokinase, urokinase, TPA and reteplase) act as thrombolytic agents by activating plasminogen to plasmin, which degrades fibrin and hence breaks up thrombi.
- *Indication:* myocardial infraction with either ST segment elevation or bundle branch block, large life threatening PE , acute non hemorrhagic CVA (<4 hrs old), acute leg ischemia (usually <14/7 with no evidence of tissue necrosis) or complex DVT (DVT with venous gangrene, ischemia or cardiopulmonary compromise or extensive DVT involving the iliac and more central veins).
- See 📖 Chapter 6 and 15 for more detailed protocols.

Vasodilators

May be required for spasm. Glyceryl trinitrate 100–200 mg boluses by intra-arterial injection are sufficient but may need an infusion of 15–20 mg/min. The BP must be monitored closely.

Medications post intervention

Aspirin (50–330 mg), with or without dipyridamol, reduces arterial re-narrowing and the incidence of re-occlusion at 6 to 12 months compared with no therapy or vitamin K antagonists. Ideally aspirin should be continued life-long.

All risk factors should continue to be managed with a continuation of the appropriate drug therapy, as described earlier in the chapter.

Carotid artery stenting

- Aspirin 70–300 mg/day.
- Clopidogrel 75 mg/day for at least 3 days prior to the CAS procedure, or a loading dose of at least 300 mg at least 6 hours prior to the procedure.

Most operators recommend that patients commence dual antiplatelet treatment

Heparin: Once arterial access has been secured, then patients should be anticoagulated, and this is usually with heparin (although some authorities suggest other agents such as bivalirudin). The usual dose is 5000 IU of heparin.

Atropine: Prior to manipulation of the carotid bifurcation an anticholinergic medication should usually be administered. Glycopyrrolate is an alternative.

Persistent hypertension following CAS should be treated. Headaches following CAS may be an indication that reperfusion injury may be imminent, necessitating the use of blood pressure lowering agents (IV nitroglycerin, nitroprussid or labetalol).

Post procedure

It is generally recommended that dual antiplatelet therapy (aspirin 70–300 mg/day, clopidogrel 75 mg/day) has to be continued for a period of 3–6 months following CAS.

Other drugs

Intravenous medications for emergency cases:

- Nitroprusside 0,25–10 µg/kg per min. (RR monitoring required).
- Glyceryl trinitrate 5–100 µg/min. within 2–5 mins.
- Esmolol (Brevibloc®) 200–500 µg/kg p/min. for 1–2 mins, followed by 50–300 µg/kg p/Min. i.v.
- Labetalol (Trandate®) 20–80 mg i.v. bolus for 5–10 mins, followed by 2 mg/min. i.v.-infusion. AE: Nausea, AV-Bloc.

Oral medications

- Nifedipine (Adalat®) 20 mg p.o., (repeat after 15–30 mins if required). AE (adverse events): delayed prolonged hypotension; in patients with aortic stenosis.
- Captopril (Lopirin®) 25 mg p.o., (repeat after 15–30 mins if required). AE: renal failure in patients with bilateral renal artery stenosis.
- Clonidine (Catapres®) 0.15 mg p.o., (repeat after 30 mins if required for a maximal dose of 0.6 mg). AE: hypotension, sedation.
- Labetalol (Trandate®) 200–400 mg p.o. (repeat after 30 mins if required). AE: bronchospasm, AV-bloc.

Sedation and analgesia

Level of sedation

The level of sedation forms a therapeutic continuum consisting of 4 stages.

Minimal (anxiolysis) sedation

Drug induced state. Patients respond normally to verbal commands.

Moderate sedation (conscious sedation)

Patients respond purposefully to verbal commons, either alone or through tactile stimulation. Patients maintain airways.

Deep sedation

A state where the patient cannot be aroused easily but responds to repeat verbal or painful stimulation. Airway maintenance may be impaired.

General anesthesia

Patient is not arousable and cannot maintain airway.

Minimal requirements of monitoring during sedation

BP, pulse, oxygen sat, ECG, and blood glucose level.

Medication used for sedation and analgesia

Hypnotic and sedative agents

The most commonly used agents are benzodiazepines, propofol, and Ketamine.

Benzodiazepines

Act on GABA receptor. Causes anxiolysis, antegrade amnesia, hypnosis, and anticonvulsant effects. No analgesic effect. Use flumazenil to reverse the effect of benzodiaepines and the effect can last up to 2 hrs. The patient must therefore be monitored for 2 hrs with flumazenil administration.

Common drugs i.e.:
- *Midazolam*.(IV/O) Short acting. Onset of action is within 2 mins. Effects last for 45–60 mins. Should be given in 1 mg increments.
- *Diazepam:* (IV, O, PR & IM) Medium acting. Onset of action 1–2mins, effect can last up to 6 hrs. Use a lipid emulsion preparation as the aqueous solution is painful at the injection site.
- *Lorazepam:* (O, IV, IM SL). Long acting. Onset of action 60–90 mins. Effect can be up to 48 hrs.

Propofol: (*IV only*) A popular induction agent. Administered in a 1–20 mg bolus. Onset of action is 60 secs. Effect can last for 3–5 mins. Better sedative effect compared to midazolam. Can cause unpredictable loss of airways and requires input from anesthesiologists for administration.

Ketamine (IV, IM, O and trasmucosally). NMDA receptor antagonist. A popular choice during pediatric interventional procedures. Produces dissociative amnesia (analgesia, amnesia, sedation with increased muscle tone which help to maintain airway). Contraindicated in patients with raised IC pressure. Onset of action within 1–2 mins. Effect can last up to 50 mins.

Analgesic agents

Broadly divided into local or systemic analgesics agents.

Systemic agents: Main categories include acetaminophine, NSAID, opioids, and nitrous oxide.

Acetaminophen: Oral. It possesses analgesic and antipyretic properties. Little anti-inflammatory effect.

- *NSAIDs:* can be further divided into salicylate or non-salicylate agents. Aspirin is a well-known salicylate derivative.
- Analgesic, antipyrectic, and anti-inflamatory effects.
- Also well-known antiplatelet agents.
- Nonsalicylate agents (ibuprofen, naproxen, diclofenac) are favoured for their analgesic and anti-inflammatory effect owing to a favourable side effect profile.
- NSAID's are contraindicated in patients with peptic ulcer, asthma, and renal failure.

Opioids

- Act on Mu, Delta, Kappa and Sigma receptors. Potent analgesics with sedative effects.
- Commonly used agents include fentanyl, morphine, sufentanil and remifentanil.
  - *Fentanyl:* Short acting. Onset of action is within 2–3 mins. Analgesic effect can last up to 60 mins. The respiratory depressant effect can last up to 4 hrs.
  - *Morphine:* Long acting agent. Onset of action is within 10 mins and effect can last for 4 hrs.
  - *Sufentanil:* Short acting. 10 times more potent than fentanyl.
  - *Remifentanil:* Rapid onset of action within 1–2 mins with short duration effect (5–7 mins). Popular choice for RFA and vertebralplasty procedures.
  - *Naloxone* is the reversal agent and repeated doses may be required in the case of long acting opioid toxicity as the duration of action is less than 90 mins.

Nitrous oxide

- A colourless inorganic gas.
- Analgesic effect at low concentration.
- Disinhibitory effect at high level.
- Administered in 50% oxygen through a mask. Onset of action is within minutes and the effect is terminated within 60 secs of removing the mask. Requires a well ventilated room.

Contrast agents

An ideal contrast agent would be easy to use, mix well with blood, have no side-effects for the patient, and be inexpensive.

Iodinated Contrast Media (ICM)

- All currently used iodinated contrast media are chemical modifications of a 2, 4, 6-tri-iodinated benzene ring.
- Classified according to their physical and chemical characteristics.
- Iodine can be easily combined with other molecules.
- By increasing the attenuation of X-rays, it is a positive contrast agent.

High-osmolality contrast media

- Tri-iodinated benzene ring with 2 organic side chains and a carboxyl group.
- The iodinated anion (diatrizoate or iothalamate) is conjugated with a cation (sodium or meglumine) giving an ionic monomer.
- The ionization at the carboxyl-cation bond makes the agent water-soluble.
- The osmolality in solution ranges from 600–2100 mOsm/kg (290 mOsm/kg human plasma).
- Ionic monomers are sub-classified by the percentage weight of the contrast agent molecule in solution (e.g. 30% or 76%).

Low-osmolality contrast media

1. Non-ionic monomers

- Contrast agent of choice because of their non-ionic nature and lower osmolality, they are less chemo-toxic than ionic monomers.
- The tri-iodinated benzene ring is made water-soluble by the addition of hydrophilic hydroxyl groups to organic side chains.
- Because there is no carboxyl group, non-ionic monomers do not ionize in solution. Therefore they have half the osmolality of ionic monomers in solution.
- They are sub-classified according to the number of milligrams of iodine in 1 ml of solution (e.g. 240, 300 or 370 mg/mL).
- Examples of common non-ionic monomers are:
  - iohexol (Omnipaque; GE Healthcare, Inc.)
  - iopamidol (Isovue; Bracco Diagnostics, Inc.)
  - ioversol (Optiray, Tyco Healthcare and Mallinckrodt, Inc.)
  - iopromide (Ultravist; Bayer Healthcare Pharmaceuticals, Inc.).

2. Ionic dimers:

- Formed from 2 ionic monomers with the elimination of 1 carboxyl group, they contain 6 iodine atoms for every 2 particles in solution.
- Concentration of 320 mgI/mL, osmolality of 600 mOsm/kg.
- Only one is commercially available:
  - ioxaglate (Hexabrix; Tyco Healthcare and Mallinckrodt, Inc.).

3. Non-ionic dimers:

- Formed from 2 joined non-ionic monomers, they contain 6 iodine atoms for every 1 particle in solution.
- For a given iodine concentration, the non-ionic dimmers have the lowest osmolality of all the contrast agents.

- Because of their high viscosity, they have limited clinical use.
- Examples of non-ionic dimers include:
  - Iotrol and iodixanol (Visipaque; Amersham Health, Inc.).

Adverse reactions to Iodinated Contrast Media (ICM)
- The incidence of any adverse reaction to ICM is 15%.
- The risk of contrast reaction is significantly less with low osmolality contrast agents than with high osmolality contrast agents and with non-ionic contrast media compared to ionic contrast media.
- As a precaution, all patients should be monitored for a minimum of 20 mins post ICM injection.
- The rooms where ICM is administered should be equipped with basic life support facilities, equipment, and drugs.

Types of adverse reactions to Iodinated Contrast Media

Idiosyncratic
- The pathogenesis involves direct cellular effects; enzyme induction; activation of complement, fibrinolytic, kinin, and other systems.
- These reactions begin within 20 mins of ICM injection and independent of the dose administered.
- They differ from true anaphylactic reactions in the following ways:
  - They are not true hypersensitivity reactions as IgE antibodies are not involved.
  - Previous sensitization is not required.
- These reactions do not recur consistently (although they may do).
- Symptoms may be:
  - Mild: urticaria, rhinorrhea, nausea/vomiting, diaphoresis, coughing, dizziness. No treatment is required.
  - Moderate: persistent vomiting, diffuse urticaria, headache, facial/laryngeal oedema, mild bronchospasm, syspesia, palpiatations, tachycardia, hypertension, abdominal cramps.
  - Severe: life threatening arrhythmias, hypotension, overt bronchospasm or laryngeal oedema, pulmonary oedema, seizures, syncope, death.
- Risks of idiosynchratic reactions:
  - Previous reaction to ionic or non-ionic ICM (increased risk of repeat reaction 3.3–6.9 times).
  - Asthma (1.2–2.5 times risk of reaction and 5–9 times more likely to be severe).
  - Food allergy (1.5–3 times more likely to have adverse reactions to ICM).

Non-idiosyncratic:
Bradycardia, hypotension, vasovagal reactions, nephropathy, extravazation, delayed reactions.
- Heightened parasympathetic activity: bradycardia, peripheral vasodilatation. Autonomic manifestations: nausea, vomiting, sphincter dysfunction.
- Nephropathy: elevation of the serum creatinine level or more than 25% of the baseline level at 1–3 days post ICM. The creatinine level usually returns to baseline in 10–14 days.
  - The incidence of contrast agent related nephropathy is estimated at 2–7%.

- Due to pre-existing haemodynamic alterations, renal vasoconstriction due to mediators such as endothelin and adenosine and direct cellular toxicity.
- Pre-existing renal insufficiency patients have 5–10 times the risk of ICM-related nephropathy.
- Patients with diabetic nephropathy are at the greatest risk and at the greatest risk of irreversible renal deterioration.
- Other conditions predisposing to ICM-related nephropathy include congestive heart failure, dehydration, concomitant use of nephrotoxic drugs (NSAID's, aminoglycosides), cirrhosis and nephrotic syndrome.
- Mannitol and furosemide have not been demonstrated to be helpful prophylactically in ICM-related nephropathy.
- IV or oral theophylline, acetylcysteine, fenoldapam or bosentan (an endothelin antagonist) may prove useful. Suggested doses of 600 mg acetylcysteine twice daily with rehydration may reduce the incidence of ICM-related nephropathy.

- Cardiovascular: Bradycardia, hypotension, due to vasovagal reaction, a direct negative inotropic effect of ICM on the myocardium, and peripheral vasodilatation. ICM can lower the ventricular arrhythmia threshold. Fluid shifts occurring due to infusion of a hyperosmolar intravascular fluid can produce intravascular hypervolaemia. Systemic hypertension and pulmonary oedema.
- Others: syncope, seizures, aggravation of phaeochromocytomas, sickle cell anaemia, hyperthyroidism, and myasthenia gravis.
- Extravasation: extravasation of ICM into soft tissues can lead to tissue damage as a direct toxic effect, or due to pressure effects such as in compartment syndrome.
- Delayed reactions: Between 30 mins and 7 days of the ICM injection.
  - These are common (14–30% patients when ionic monomers are used, 8–10% of patients when non-ionic monomers are used).
  - Symptoms include flu-like syndrome with fatigue, weakness, upper respiratory tract congestion, fevers, nausea, diarrhea, abdominal pain, dizziness, and headache. Less frequent manifestations include pruritis, polyarthropathy, and depression.
  - Increased incidence and severity in cancer patients treated with interleukin-2 immunotherapy
  - Lactic acidosis may be induced by increased tissue levels of metformin post ICM-administration. Metformin is excreted renally and ICM-administration may lead to delayed excretion. Metformin should be discontinued for 48 hours after ICM administration and resumed in the absence of renal dysfunction.
  - Pregnancy: in vitro experiments have demonstrated a mutagenic effect of ICM but no teratogenic effects have been documented in vivo. ICM does cross the placenta and can potentially produce transient fetal hypothyroidism.

Recommended Prophylactic Regime
- Methyl-prednisolone 32 mg orally 12 and 2 hrs prior to the study;
or
- Prednisolone 50 mg orally 13 hrs, 7 hrs and 1 hr before the study.

- In addition, anti-histamines such as diphenhydramine 50 mg orally 1 hr prior to the study, cimetidine 300 mg orally 1 hr before the study may be prescribed.

Barium sulphate

Commonly used in the digestive tract; it is usually swallowed or administered as an enema or prior to gastrostomy in order to opacify the colon.

Microbubbles

- A new class of contrast agents used mainly as an intravascular contrast media for US.
- Can also be instilled into the bladder to look for ureteric reflux.
- They are 1–7 mm in diameter and consist of an stabilizing shell (made of denatured albumin, surfactants or phospholipids) and contain gas (usually air or perfluro gas).
- Examples include Sono Vue® and perflutren (Definity®).

Indication

Used in assessing renal artery stenosis, assessing difficult hepatic and portal vascular examination, identifying liver, breast, and renal lesion before and after biopsy/radiofrquency ablation. It is safe in patients with renal failure. **Its use is contraindicated in patients with unstable ischemic heart disease**

Carbon dioxide

A cheap, non-allergic and non nephrotoxic contrast agent. Pure medical graded CO_2 from a closed delivery system must be used in order to avoid air embolism.

Indication

- Patients with a history of severe contrast reaction who cannot be investigated with MRI or US.
- To identify the portal vein in difficult TIPS procedure, hepatic wedge venography, guiding TIPS and the detection of GI hemorrhage and endoleaks.
- Do not use intrarterial carbon dioxide above the diaphragm owing to the increased risk of neurotoxicity.
- Also avoid the use in patients with right to left intracardiac shunt.
- A large volume can result in vapour lock.

MRI contrast agents

MRI contrast agents are mainly categorized as extracellulalr agents, reticuloendothelail agents, hepatobiliary agents, blood pool agents, and combined agents.

Extracellular agents

- GD based agent (Magnevest (gadopentate dimeglumine: Schering AG), Dotarem (Gadoterate meglumine: Guerbet), Omniscan (gadodiamide, Nycomed), ProHance (gadobutrol, Scheing AG) and OptiMARK (gadoversetamide, Mallinkrodt).
- They shorten the T1 and T2 relaxation time and result in signal enhancement of T1 weights imaging and signal loss at T2 and STIR sequence.

- Nephrotoxic at high doses and avoid using high doses in patients with significant renal failure.
- There is also a high risk of nephrogenic systemic sclerosis (NSF) with the use of gadodiamide (Ominiscan™), gadopentate dimeglumine (Magnevist®) and gadoversetamide (OptiMark®) in patients with pre exisiting renal failure.

Gadolinium Chelate for DSA

The physical properties of gadolinium chelate which contribute to its suitability as a contrast agent include:

- Gadolinium (Z=64) has a higher atomic number than iodine (Z=53), a positive contrast agent.
- Higher k edge (50 KeV) than iodine (33 KeV). Allows imaging at a higher kilovolt peak without loss of contrast. Imaging at 96 kVp results in better image quality with a lower radiation dose than the 70–80 kVp used with iodinated contrast media.
- Free gadolinium is toxic, but several preparations of gadolinium chelates are available for routine use as an MRI contrast agent.
- Gadoluinm chelates are excreted renaly with an elimination half-life of 1.5 hours with normal renal function.
- All gadolinium chelates are liquid agents.
- Several different gadolinium chelates in clinical use. Differences in their chemical structures lead to variations in the likelihood of dissociation.
- Cyclic molecules, containing Gd3+ ion within a cavity in their structure, are less likely to dissociate than linear molecules. *Ionic cyclic chelates (Dotarem) are the least likely to release free Gd3+.*

Indications for use of gadolinium chelate as a contrast agent

- Known or suspected severe allergy to iodinated contrast media.
- Mild-moderate renal impairment including renal transplant recipients.

Contra-indications

- Severe renal impairment (GFR <30 mL/min/1.73m2), due to the risk of nephrogenic systemic fibrosis.
- Gadolinium Chelate for DSA

Patient preparation

- Standard preparation for catheter angiography.
- No pre-medication with steroids or fluid bolus required.

Technique

- Conventional catheter placement under fluoroscopy.
- Acquired using digital subtraction; standard gadolinium chelates less radio-opaque than iodinated contrast media and non-subtracted images provide insufficient image quality.
- The examination must be tailored to allow sufficient image acquisition without exceeding the maximum permissible dose (see below).

Maximum dose

- Small doses are administered routinely intra-venously in MRI imaging. There is limited data on maximum dose administration for intra-arterial use but a recommended upper limit is 0.3–0.4 mmol/kg body weight.

- This limits the total dose for a 70 kg patient to 42–56 mL (21–28 mg) requiring careful tailoring of the examination. A 1:1 dilution of saline increases the total volume available allowing small vessels to be imaged but with lower radio-opacity.

Adverse reaction
- <1% of patients undergoing administration of gadolinium chelates (for MRI imaging)
- Include nausea, headaches.
- Anaphylaxis (1 in 100,000–500,000).
- Association with nephrogenic systemic fibrosis.

Anti-peristaltic drugs
- Useful for obtaining good mesenteric angiograms and for some bowel related procdures.
- Buscopan® 40 mg to maximum of 160 mg IV. Caution glaucoma, dysrythmias, tachycardia and heart failure. Monitor ECG, Pulse and BP.
- Glucogan 1 mg, Caution in patients with Insulinoma and Phaeochromoctoma.

Anti-emetics
There is a wide range of good drugs available for IV use in the BNF.

Equipment

The key to interventional radiology is knowing which equipment is available and in which circumstances and how to use it. The following are the most commonly used.

Needles

One part or two part.

Single part needles (Figure 3.1) only require a puncture of the anterior wall, but can result in subintimal entry of the guidewire if the bevel is not completely within the lumen. It is therefore vital that there is a good pulsatile blood flow from the hub before introducing the guidewire.

Two part needles (Figure 3.2) are very simple to use but require a double wall puncture, i.e. both the front and back wall of the artery. The sharp central trochar is removed and the outer metal cannula slowly withdrawn until there is a good blood flow. This is said to have a reduced risk of dissection but has the disadvantage of a potential hemorrhage from the posterior wall puncture, particularly for thrombolysis.

An 18 gauge Chiba needle or 14F Abbocatheter is used for deep vessels in obese patients.

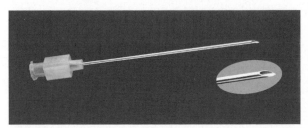

Figure 3.1 Single part needle with a simple bevel.

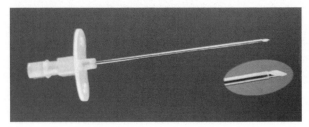

Figure 3.2 Two part needle has an inner trochar which is removed following puncture leaving a blunt atraumatic end. © Cook.

Micropuncture kit

This has a 22 gauge single part needle with a 0.18 wire. It is generally used for access to small vessels, i.e. radial, tibial, etc.

Guidewires

(see Figure 3.3)

The main function of guidewires is for the support of catheters (non steerable) and for help in cannulation of branch vessels (particularly steerable wires).

- Always advance the guidewire under fluoroscopy so as not to cause inadvertent dissection (looping of stiff wire) or branch vessel damage.
- If the wire sticks check why! If the wire does not pass through the access needle this means either the needle is against or in the wall (either posterior or anterior). This may be because of severe disease and if advancing the needle slightly or some cases retracting the needle does not give good back bleeding or the wire still cannot be advanced, try slightly higher or lower in the CF (see 📖 Chapter 5).
- Never use hydrophilic wires directly through the needle as the coating can shear off and embolize.
- A good length of wire should be within the artery or beyond the target lesion/vessel before trying to advance a catheter
- When advancing catheters over the wire, the wire must remain fixed and should literally be pinned by the assistant to the table otherwise there will be kinking and buckling of the wire and catheter.
- With steerable wires a combination of curved catheter and wire will easily allow tortuous segments to be negotiated and the most awkward cannulations can be performed. For small distal vessels micro-catheters and wires will be required.
- Tricks with wires. Standard J wires usually come with a little straightner. However it is very simple to grip the wire in your hand, and grip with the middle to little finger against the thenar eminence while pushing forward with the wire held in the index finger and thumb, which effectively pulls the curve straight for introduction into the catheter hub.

There are literally dozens of different types. They are measured in fractions of an inch in circumference, i.e. 0.14, 0.18, 0.35 or 0.38. The standard length is 145 cm but can go up to >400 cm .

Thinner wires, i.e. 0.14/0.18, etc. are used generally to allow the use of smaller profile catheters, i.e. micro-catheters for embolization /equipment including balloons.

Length is chosen so as to allow catheter exchange. There may be a hydrophilic coating to make them more steerable through tortuous arteries or tight stenosis, i.e. Terumo (Terumo Corporation Japan) or Road Runner (Cooks, UK). They need to be kept wet or they become very sticky. They are not generally reliable in supporting delivery for bulky devices or large French size catheters.

Stiffness depends on thickness and differences in material, i.e. stainless steel, Nitinol, etc.

There are grades of increased rigidity of wires which markedly increases support for delivering bulky catheter and delivery systems but reduces flexibility and the ability of the wires to negotiate complex anatomy.

- Standard wires: 3 mm, 5 mm or 15 mm J or straight commonly used for initial puncture.
- Soft wires: Bentson for crossing stensosis or tortuous seg ments and pushing coils. Will flop through moderate stenosis with gentle pushing.
- Moderate stiffness: Heavy duty or Amplatz stiff.
- Very stiff: Amplatz superstiff or ultrastiff and Myre wires.
- Extremely stiff: Lunderquist (like a coat hanger wire, almost as stiff!).
- Steerable wires: Terumo/Roadrunner for crossing tight stenosis or tortuous vessels. Stiff Terumo combines support and steerablility.
- Graduated wire which increases in stiffness from proximal to distal, i.e. TAD/Jindo which goes from a 0.18 diameter 4 cm floppy tip to an 0.35 rigid shaft, useful in renal or mesenteric stenting.
- 0.18 wires, i.e. V18 control wire for use with smaller vessels and catheters/balloons with a floppy tip but stiff main shaft..
- Micro wires for microcatheters or small F size balloons, of which there are many varying in size from 0.14 and up, varying stiffness with or without hydrophilic coating including Terumo wires.

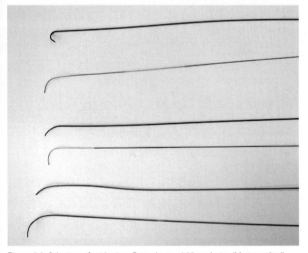

Figure 3.3 Selection of guidewires. From the top 0.35mm J wire (Merit medical), 0.18 V18 control wire (Boston Scientific), curved Terumo wire (Terumo Corporation), Jindo wire (Cordis UK), Amplatz superstiff (Boston Scientific) and Lunderquist exchange wire (Cook UK).

PinVise

(see Figure 3.4)

Very useful for gripping the wire for torque control particularly when using hydrophilic wires. There are different sizes for 0.14 or 0.35 wires.

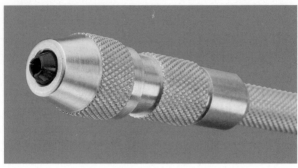

Figure 3.4 Pinvise hub which by rotating grips a wire for torque control. © Cook.

Catheters

Measured in French size (F). One French is equivalent to 0.33 of a mm, i.e. 3F = 1 mm in diameter. Typically most modern catheters are 5F or less.

Smaller catheters make smaller entry holes and limit bleeding complications, while larger French sizes give more torque control (i.e. steerability).

Modern catheters are made of plastic and are generally braided (re-inforced internally in the wall to increase strength. They may also have a slippery coating to reduce resistance and improve maneuverability.

Diagnostic catheters have multiple side holes in addition to an end hole to allow rapid injection of large volumes of contrast medium. The most commonly used are pigtails (Figure 3.5) in shape in order to avoid injection of contrast into the vessel wall by an end hole jet, but they can be straight or a variety of other shapes depending on site, i.e. for cardiac/ pulmonary or peripheral vascular use.

Flow rates are determined by the lumen size , number of side holes, pressure of injection, and length. Typical flow rates are:

- 3F 6–8 mls/second.
- 4F 16–18 mls/second.
- 5F 20–25 mls/seond, etc.

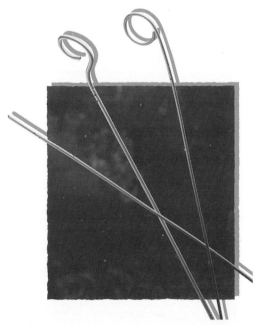

Figure 3.5 Selection of flush angiographic catheters. Pigtail most frequently used.
© Cordis

Preshaped selective catheters

These are used to help to change guidewire direction, cannulate branch vessels, and help negotiate complex lesions, i.e. tortuousity, stenosis, and angulation of branch vessels (Figure 3.6).

There are a huge number of cardiac and peripheral catheters; the following are the most commonly used catheters:

Use: When steering catheters it is vital that the catheter is rotated at the puncture site and the distal end to gain maximum torque.

- Cobra (C1–3 Figure 3.7) (selection of renal, mesenteric vessels, occasionally crossing the iliac bifurcation in young females in particular, selecting the SFA in difficult antegrade punctures, etc.). The catheter may be pulled down or pushed up to engage the branch and advanced over the wire thereafter.
- Sidewinders or Simmonds (1–3 Figure 3.8) (Most useful in cannulating mesenteric vessels, but also crossing the iliac bifurcation, selecting arch vessels, hepatic veins from a groin approach, etc.). Used very differently than other catheters. It is formed by pushing the catheter, without the wire, into the arch, ideally with the end in the left subclavian and twisting 360 degrees or more until a shepherd's crook type shape is formed. It then needs to come down slowly avoiding branch vessels on the way down (Figure 3.8).

TIPS:

Having a guidewire just 3–4 cm out the catheter tip as it is withdrawn will prevent inadvertent wire entry into branches.
To advance the catheter into a branch the catheter is pulled into it and then the wire advanced into the vessel to give support and then the catheter advanced over it.

- SoS OMNI (very similar to Sidewinders but with a smaller head, do not need to form in the arch, also the best catheter for retrograde to antegrade conversion).
- Multipurpose (selective cannulation of infra-inguinal vessels).
- Headhunter (cannulation of arch vessels and used for contralateral puncture approach).
- Bernstein (top left) or vertebral (top right) (Figure 3.9). Selection of arch vessels and distal tibial vessel stenosis.
- Renal curve (bottom) or double curve (Figure 3.9) used for crossing the bifurcation or cannulation of renal vessels.

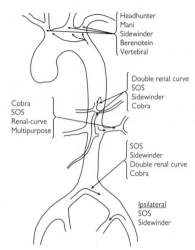

Figure 3.6 Commonly used catheters in different territories of the vascular tree.

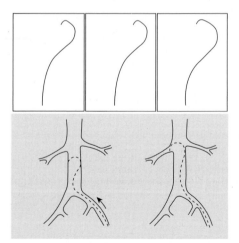

Figure 3.7 Cobra catheters C1-3 showing increasing size of the head and curve. C2 most commonly used by pushing or pulling down into the vessel. This is often sufficient to perform an hand injection angiogram. If a more selective position required., a guidwire is advanced into the selective vessel and when sufficient wire in to the vessel i.e 7–8cm the catheter is advanced for more selective position. © Terumo.

Tip: rotating the catheter as you advance helps it track along the wire.

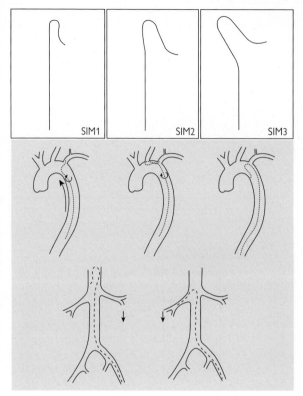

Figure 3.8 Sidewinder catheters (SIMS) 1-3. Initially when introduced over the wire it is relatively straight. Form a hook shape by advancing into the arch of the aorta, remove the guidwire, engage into the subclavian artery and rotate 360 degrees, while advancing forms hook shape.

TIP: Sometimes it is twisted/knotted, this can be undone by introducing a wire out of the tip.

To engage a vessel it is pulled down into it until the catheter almost starts to straighten. This is sufficient to get good angiographic pictures, even with a pump.

If need to go further, then advance a guidewire 6–7cm into the vessel and advance catheter.

Tip: Sometimes rotating the catheter as you advance helps prevent the hook reforming and pulling the wire back out.

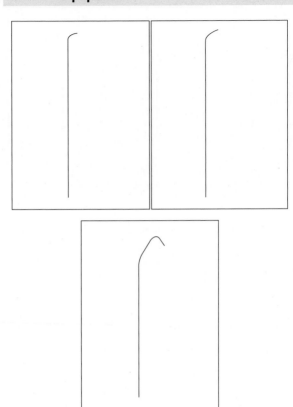

Figure 3.9 Vertebral, Berenstein and renal curve catheters. © Terumo.

Sheaths

These are used in the vast majority of interventional procedures. They consist of an inner dilater and outer sheath with an haemostatic valve. They are introduced as for catheters over the wire and then the inner dilater is then removed and the sideport flushed with heparinized saline regularly to prevent thrombus formation.

They vary from 4–30 French and 11–90 cm in length. A 4F catheter will allow the passage of 4F catheters and below and so on. This allows catheters to be easily changed while maintaining haemostasis and also contrast injection with the wire in place. It allows selective access from the femoral to branch vessels all the way to the arch, i.e. renals, mesenteric, carotids, etc.

Re-enforced sheaths with braiding in the wall to prevent kinking (Figure 3.11) are useful in tortuous anatomy and prevent kinking and allow for better control of catheters

Balkan or other curved sheaths are used for access to a contralateral femoral artery.

Disadvantages. The external diameter is at least 1F bigger and for re-inforced sheaths this can be 2–3F.

Needs constant flushing and may clot. Make sure that the sheath is not kinked.

TIPS:

Aspirate with a 50ml syringe if this fails. Exchange for another carefully over a wire, ideally with simultaneous aspiration of the side arm. Aspirating and turning the tap off immediately will maintain aspiration pressure.

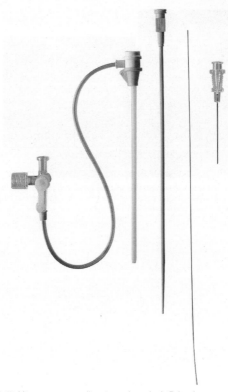

Figure 3.10 Micropuncture needle, wire, and standard 6F sheath.

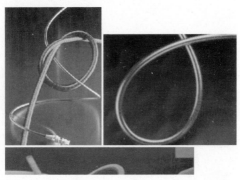

Figure 3.11 Arrowflex sheath, which is specially reinforced so it can take very toruos segments and still allow passage of a guidewire. Also used to cross the bifurcation or access into renal arteries. © Arrow.

Guiding catheters

(see Figure 3.12)

Used to give stable selective access to branch vessels and allow exchange of catheters/stents with ease and opacify branch vessels. Sizes vary from 5–10F and lengths of over 100 cm.

TIPS:

They are also useful for aspiration of thrombus in vessels. They are used in conjunction with Tuohy-Bohrst (Figure 3.13) or removable haemostatic valve (Figure 3.14) and effectively gives you a sheath with a smaller external diameter. Remember that the external diameter of the guiding catheter is the French size, as opposed to sheaths where the French size refers to the maximum diameter of the catheter that can be passed.

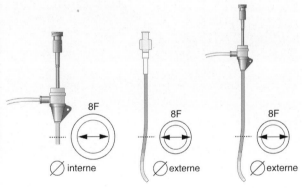

Figure 3.12 Shows difference between sheathes and guiding catheters i.e. and 8F sheath will allow passage of a 8f external diameter catheter, including guiding catheter. An 8F guiding catheter will allow 6F systems or below but will pass through a 6F sheath. © Cordis.

Tuohy-Bohrst

(see Fig 3.13):

This is a Y shaped device which has a haemostatic valve on one limb and a tap on the other. This allows smaller wires or catheters to be used in larger catheters, i.e. 0.18 wire in a 0.35 lumen as well as allowing simultaneous flushing or contrast injection.

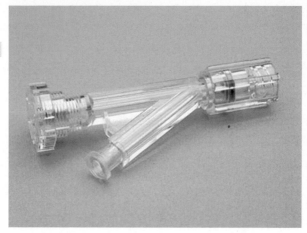

Figure 3.13 Tuohy-Bohrst. © Cook.

Removable haemostatic valve

(see Figure 3.14)

This is very useful for converting guiding catheters effectively into sheaths and during clot aspiration. The sheath can be removed in order to get all of the clotting out of the catheter.

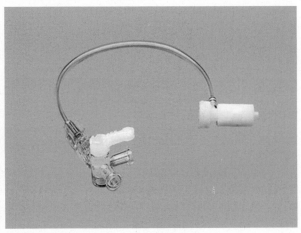

Figure 3.14 Removable haemostatic valve. © Cook.

Microcatheters

Microferret (Cook UK), Progreat (Terumo corporation, Japan), etc.1.8–3F catheters which will pass through standard 0.35 lumen selective catheters. They are used with microwires for emboliztion of distal small vessels, i.e. GI bleeders or type II endoleaks.

TIPS:

Always use Tuohy–Borst ideally with pressurized saline to flush between the inner and outer catheters in order to stop the sticking of catheters.

Stent

Balloon expandable	Original stents, useful for flush common iliac lesions and accurate placement and fully expanding stentgrafts (Figure 3.15)
Self expanding	Most common modern stents (Figure 3.16). Usually very simple deployment by smoothly retracting the outer sheath back on the inner core. Some have special mechanisms to help in slow accurate release which effectively do the same as above
Drug eluting	Mainly balloon expandable, used in cardiac limited peripheral use
Stentgrafts	Balloon expandable or self expanding. Mainly used to treat aneurysm and rupture (Figure 3.17). Should be available in all departments
Balloons	0.14 system and monorail systems have lower profiles and go through smaller sheaths. Burst pressure decreases with increase in balloon size. Virtually all are semi-compliant, i.e. will increase slightly in size above stated level with increasing pressure beyond their optimum (usually 6 atm)
Standard (Figure 3.18a)	Used for most peripheral angioplasty (Burst pressure 12–15 atm)
Monorail (Figure 3.18b)	Most commonly used in cardiac, carotid or renal angioplasty allows rapid exchange and smaller sheath size
High pressure	For resistant lesions, i.e. Venous strictures or Intimal hyperplasia (burst pressure 15–30 atm depending on size)
Cutting balloons (Figure 3.19)	Boston Scientific, UK. As for high pressure. Only come in 1–2 cm lengths and up to 8 mm diameter. Use standard balloon if necessary to increase diameter of lumen. Don't use cutting balloon after standard balloon due to risk of rupture
Inflation devices: (Figure 3.20)	Although a simple syringe and tap will allow balloon inflation, these should be used to give more controlled dilatation and avoid rupture

Retrieval devices	Used for retrieval foreign bodies most commonly catheter fragments, coils, stents, pacing leads or re-orientation of lines (see 📖 Chapter 21)
Snares	Varies types, i.e. single loop Amplatz Gooseneck, Ensare, Trisnare – 3 loops at right angles
Graspers	
Baskets	

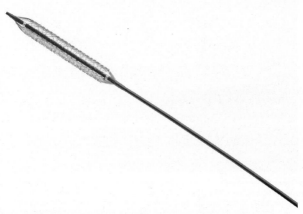

Figure 3.15 Balloon expandable stent. These come in 12-80mm lengths and can be expanded up to 10-12mm for standard stents. Usually pre-mounted on the appropriate balloon. Large Palmaz stents can be expanded to 30mm, but they do start to shorten as they are stretched beyond their intended size. Need sheath size 1-2 F larger than the balloon size. © Boston.

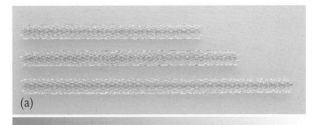

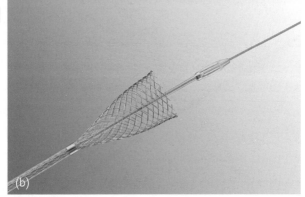

Figure 3.16 (a) Selection of selfexpanding stents giving constant radial force and expand up to predetermined size unlike balloon expandable. (b) The technique to release is simple, the outer sheath is gradually withdrawn to expose the stent. Most cannot be recovered once release started (Wall stents can be easily re-covered to a point) however they can be withdrawn if only 20-30% of the stent is released. Nitinol stents shorten minimally, wall stents shorten up to 40% and difficult to predict precisely. © Boston.

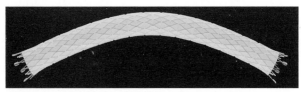

Figure 3.17 Self expanding covered stentgraft for aneurysms and acute rupture (Fluency Bard uk). There are also balloon expandable stentgrafts (Jomed/Atrium). © Bard.

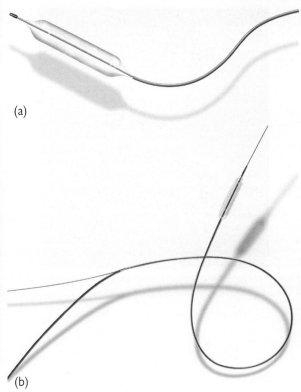

(a)

(b)

Figure 3.18 (a) Standard 0.35 Balloon. (b) Monorail balloon, often uses 0.14 wire which comes out near the balloon itself. Allow the balloons to be made smaller, poorer tracing however. © Cordis.

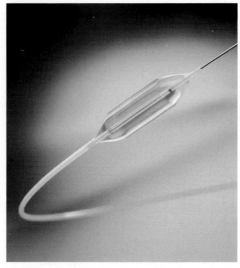

Figure 3.19 Cutting balloons come in 1-2cm length up to 8mm and go through a 7F sheath. © Boston.

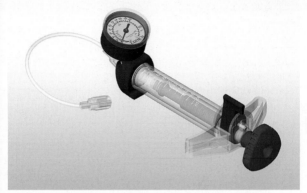

Figure 3.20 Inflation device for controlled balloon expansion. © Cook.

Imaging

Imaging should be accurate and influence treatment decisions with minimal risk and discomfort to patients.

Non-invasive imaging

Non-invasive assessment of peripheral vascular disease includes:
- Clinical assessment of peripheral pulses and measurement of ankle-brachial pressure index (ABPI).
- Imaging: duplex, magnetic resonance angiography, computerized tomography angiography.

Arterial duplex scanning

Advantages
- Non-invasive.
- Cheap.
- No side effects.
- Highly sensitive (88%) and specific (96%) for the detection of significant disease (>50% stenosis) in peripheral arteries.

Disadvantages
- Time consuming.
- Operator dependent.
- Difficulties in the aorto-iliac segments due to body habitus and bowel gas.
- Inaccuracies due to calcification.

Indications
- Non-invasive imaging of peripheral arterial system (native vessels).
- Non-invasive imaging of iliac arteries prior to intervention.
- Surveillance of peripheral arterial grafts (autologous vein and synthetic).
- Screening and surveillance of abdominal aortic aneurysms.

Technique for examination of native peripheral arterial system
- Position patient with the head elevated to 20 degrees and externally rotate the patient's leg.
- Select the appropriate examination pre-set.
- B-mode scanning: transverse plane over the abdomen to identify the aorta and vena cava. Firm pressure is required. Rotate the transducer to align in the longitudinal plane of the iliac arteries (Figure 4.1) or start from the groin to identify the common femoral artery and vein overlying the head of the femur and go retrogradely and then down the leg for the infra-inguinal vessels. The latter has the advantage of displacing bowel gas out of the pelvis.

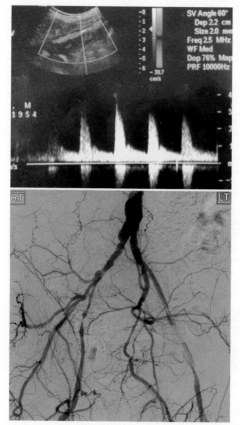

Figure 4.1 Duplex of the right external iliac artery and corresponding angiogram. There is colour aliasing, high velocities at almost 4 meters per second, with more than trebelling of velocities compared to the adjacent segments.

- Colour Doppler is then selected. The flow should show a slight reversal in diastole.
- The Doppler gate is then selected and the angle bar adjusted so it lies along the line of flow (**vital for accurate assessment, angle of insonation must be <60 degrees**). A spectral Doppler trace is obtained and a peak systolic velocity measured from the trace.

- Standard technique is to obtain spectral traces in the Aorta, iliacs, proximal, mid and distal SFA (Figure 4.2) as well as in areas of colour aliasing.
- The patient is then turned onto his side and the popliteal artery and trifurcation is examined from the back of the knee. The crural vessels can be assessed from the ankle up.

> **TIPS:**
>
> **Heavy calcification:** Try obliquing the probe to get a small window for Doppler assessment. If short segment of disease assessment of Doppler velocities just above and below may be sufficient.
>
> **Bowel gas:** Try scanning from the groin up, bowel cleansing or try again another day.
>
> **Sono CT:** on newer machines to reduce artefacts.
>
> **Ultrasound contrast:** Increase accuracy and reduce scanning times.
>
> **Note**: In healthy peripheral limb arteries a triphasic waveform is obtained. Will vary in other territories. With increasing age and vessel hardening this may become biphasic. Monophasic usually means significant stenosis. If unable to assess iliac directly a triphasic waveform in the CF usually means no significant disease.
>
> **Beware that in 10% of patients a triphasic waveform is seen in CF arteries despite upstream iliac stenosis.**

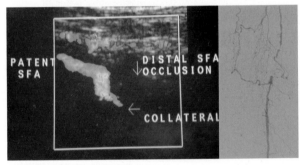

Figure 4.2 Duplex of the distal SFA with corresponding angiogram showing an occlusion with absence of flow of the colour Doppler and large collateral.

Assessing a suspected stenosis

- Spectral broadening (filling in of the spectral trace under the curve) occurs where there is turbulent flow and or flow reversal (usually related to stenosis).
- Colour Doppler imaging highlights potential stenoses as areas of aliasing.

- Aliasing occurs when there is insufficient sampling of the Doppler signal (Nyquist limit) resulting in incorrect estimation of the Doppler shift frequency and is displayed as flow in the opposite direction.
- On colour Doppler the colour trace will wrap round from red – yellow – green – blue, or vice-versa.
- Spectral Doppler is then used to assess these areas and measure flow velocities.
- In an area of aliasing, increase the PRF gradually, a focal area of maximal aliasing can be highlighted corresponding to maximal velocity.
- The Peak Systolic Velocity (PSV) is then measured from this site.
- A second spectral Doppler trace is then recorded from the nearest normal proximal segment of the artery and a second peak systolic velocity measured.
- The ratio of peak systolic velocities between the site of aliasing and the normal vessel is calculated.
- A ratio of >2–2.5, i.e. diameter reduction of >50% or an area reduction of >75%, indicates a significant stenosis.
- Other techniques for assessing stenoses involve measurement of end diastolic velocity, number of phases in Doppler waveform and degree of spectral broadening.

The principles of Doppler effect and ultrasound

- The ultrasound transducer (probe) sends out an echo of a specific frequency.
- Echos returning back from stationary tissues return at the same frequency.
- Echos returning from moving objects, such as flowing blood, do so at a higher or lower frequency, depending on whether the object is moving toward or away from the transducer.
- The ultrasound scanner detects the change in frequency and calculates the velocity of blood flow using the Doppler frequency shift equation:

$$ft - fr = (2v\, ft\, \cos A)/c$$

where
- v = velocity of blood
- ft = transmitted frequency
- fr = received frequency
- A = angle of insonation
- c = speed of sound

Ultrasound machine optimization

- Many newer machines will have automatic pre-set buttons to guide the operator.
- Transducer Frequency: the optimal range for most peripheral arterial scanning is 5.0–7.5 MHz. This will provide adequate depth, range and image resolution. Linear array scan head (frequency range 4.0–9.0 MHz) allows beam steering.
- B-mode gain: The image gain should be set so the lumen of the normal vessel appears black. A moderate to high contrast image provides a better visualization of the anechoic vessel against the surrounding echogenic soft tissues.
- Pulse repetition frequency (PRF): The colour Doppler PRF should be set in the 3000–4000 Hz range in order to sample normal arterial flow.

This will show the centre of the lumen at the upper end of the colour range without producing aliasing.

- Colour gain: This should be set to a level where it completely fills the lumen of a normal vessel without colour 'bleeding' into the surrounding tissues.
- High pass or wall filter: this filters out the high-amplitude, low-frequency Doppler signal produced by vessel wall movement. **If set too high, it may alter the shape of the spectral Doppler wave form.**

Carotid duplex

The duplex of carotid and vertebral arteries is used by the majority of centers for the assessment of patients with suspected significant carotid stenosis in order to select patients for possible intervention. Good technique and training is vital.

Key points
- ICA is a low impedance vessel with flow during systole and diastole.
- 0%–49% stenosis PSV <125 cm/s with increasing spectral broadening with disease.
- 50–79% stenosis PSV >125cm/s with marked spectral broadening during sytole.
- 80–99% stenosis PSV >125cm/s and EDV >140cm/s with marked spectral broadening
- Using PSV of >210 cm/s and EDV of 110cm/s gives accuracy of 93%, sensitivity of 96% and specificity of 91% for >70% stenosis.
- No technique or parameter is 100% accurate.

NASCET criteria for stenosis compares stenotic segment to normal ICA beyond.

ECST criteria compare the stenotic diameter to the estimated diameter at the same level without disease giving a tighter % stenosis.

Computerized tomography angiography (CTA)

Advantages
- Non-invasive.
- Highly sensitive (91%) and specific (91%) for the detection of significant disease. Short stenoses may be missed.
- Reproducible.
- New techniques and post-processing techniques allow reformatted images to be displayed in multi-planar and 3D views.
- Excellent visualization of adjacent non-vascular structures.
- Better than DSA for assessing eccentric stenosis and occlusion length.
- Spatial resolution is the same in both axial and longitudinal views because each voxel is isotropic (cube not rectangle).

Disadvantages
- Requires ionizing radiation.
- Requires intravenous iodinated contrast media (see 📖 p.14).
- Resolution is inferior to conventional angiography, short stenosis may be missed, differentiation of tight stenosis versus occlusions difficult and no information on flow.
- Caution is needed in the interpretation of reconstructed images as errors in data manipulation can lead to incorrect diagnoses. Reference should be made to axial source images.
- Calcification may lead to misinterpretation of reconstructions (blooming artifact).
- Artifacts from metallic prostheses and oral iodinated contrast may lead to difficulties in interpretation.
- Timing of image acquisition in relation to contrast administration is crucial: delayed imaging results in venous enhancement, early imaging results in non-opacified arteries.

Scan Parameters
- Essentially two techniques:
  - High resolution of smaller volumes (e.g. renal arteries).
  - High speed for larger volumes (e.g. aortic aneurysms, peripheral arteries).
- The narrower the slice collimation, the better the spatial resolution.
- An array of detectors is used so that more than one slice is acquired per rotation of the gantry.
- The minimum number of detectors for adequate angiography is four, but 16 or 32 are optimal. 64-detector CT scanners are the fastest currently available and are ideal for cardiac imaging.
- The gantry rotation time is typically 500 milliseconds.

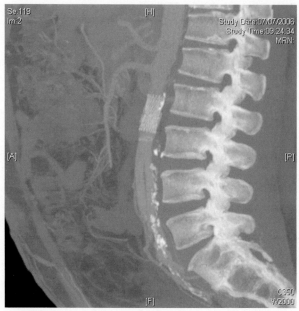

Figure 4.3 Sagittal reconstruction of a CTA showing a Palmaz stent used to treat a aortic stenosis.

- The combination of fast rotation and multi-detector acquisition means that large body volumes can be imaged during peak arterial enhancement.

Contrast Delivery

- The aim of scanning is to acquire images during peak arterial enhancement. This can be done in one of three ways:
  - Peripheral contrast injection results in a plateau contrast concentration that has to be maintained throughout the scan. The faster the scanner, the lower the volume of contrast required.
  - Injection rate may be constant or biphasic (initial high injection rate to achieve dense enhancement followed by a slower rate to maintain the plateau.
  - Bolus tracking:
    - A region of interest (ROI) is placed within the aorta on a test scan and the rate of enhancement tracked by serial scanning at that level. The scan is triggered at a pre-determined level (usually set at T12, threshold of 125HU for abdominal aortic scanning).
    - Test bolus: a test bolus of contrast is administered and repeated images of a target vessel acquired. The delay is calculated.

Patient Preparation for CTA

- No oral iodinated contrast. Water can be useful when imaging visceral vessels.
- Check for history of allergies, diabetes and renal impairment (see 📖 p.14)
- Adequate venous access to allow high flow contrast injections delivered via a pump. Flow rates of 3–5 mls per second require a pink or green cannula. A right arm antecubital vein is preferred.
- The injection site should be observed for possible extravasation.

Technique

- A bolus of iodinated contrast medium (120–150 mls or 350 mg/mls of iodine) is delivered via a pump injector through a peripheral intravenous cannula (4–5 mls per second). Use saline flush at the end.
- The bolus is tracked as it opacifies the vascular bed.
- Images are acquired during peak arterial enhancement.
- Multi-detector CT allows continuous rapid acquisition of images at the patient is moved rapidly through the gantry.
- Large anatomical areas may be imaged in 20–30 secs, reducing artifacts and improving spatial resolution. With 64 and above slices, there is a risk of outrunning the bolus and a delay may be needed.
- Slice thickness is determined by the thickness of the detector elements, rather than beam collimation, allowing slices of less than 1 mm in thickness.
- Image analysis is best performed on a dedicated workstation with appropriate software for image manipulation in order to reconstruct angiographic images.

Magnetic resonance angiography (MRA)

MRA has advanced rapidly and is now the most accurate non-invasive technique in the assessment of arteries in PVD.

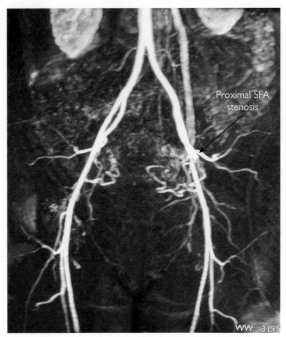

Proximal SFA stenosis

Figure 4.4 MRA of the aorto-iliac arteries showing a left external iliac artery stenosis.

Advantages

- Non-invasive.
- No ionizing radiation.
- Highly sensitive (95%) and specific (97%) for the detection of significant disease.
- Reproducible.
- Can detect eccentric stenoses, not well visualized on IADSA.
- Post-processing techniques, including subtraction, allow images to be displayed in multi-planar and 3D views.

Disadvantages

- Intolerance due to claustrophobia may be a problem in some patients (10%).
- Contra-indications: intracranial clips, implantable defibrillators and pacemakers.
- Over-estimation of the degree of stenosis.

- Cannot detect arterial calcification.
- Inaccuracies due to calcification/metallic artifact. This precludes assessment of in-stent stenoses.
- Patients with significant renal impairment (GFR <30 mLs/min) should not receive ionic linear chelates or non-ionic cyclic chelates unless it is regarded as clinically essential because of the risk of Nephrogenic systemic fibrosis (please refer to the section on Gadolinium Chelates in Renal Impairment above).

Technique

- Contrast enhanced MRA has virtually replaced 3DTOF.
- Fast 3D-spoiled-gradient-echo MR imaging sequences with minimum repetition time and echo time, with flip angles ranging from 25 to 50 degrees.
- Intravenous gadolinium chelate is administered using an automatic injector as a bolus at rates ranging from 0.5–4 mL/s I concentrations ranging from 0.05–0.3 mmol/kg.
- Timing is important; the best images are obtained when acquisition of the central portion of the k-space corresponds with the maximum concentration of contrast material in the vessel of interest, generating a high signal by means of T1 shortening of blood.
- There should be a good match between the duration of the contrast material bolus and the length of the 3D-sequence: rapid variation in the vascular concentration of contrast during acquisition of the central portion of the k-space generates significant artifacts.

Timing

- Bolus timing:
  - First a pre-contrast 3D-data-set is acquired. This serves as a final check that the volume has been positioned correctly and also tests the patient's breath-holding ability.
  - 1–2 mL of gadolinium chelate is injected along with saline solution as a flush, and the vessel of interest is scanned approximately once per second.
  - The travel time for the bolus can be directly observed and then used to calculate the correct scan delay.
  - Residual contrast material in the renal collecting systems from the test bolus may obscure branch renal artery vessels and is a potential disadvantage of using bolus timing techniques.
  - Gadolinium chelate is administered (0.15–0.2 mmol/kg at 2 mL/sec), and the arterial-phase breath-hold sequence is performed. This is followed immediately by two additional acquisitions with minimal inter-sequence delay, providing venous phase scans.
- Other timing methods:
  - Fluoroscopic triggering and automated triggering, in which the vessel of interest is continuously scanned.
  - When the gadolinium chelate bolus is directly observed or the signal intensity reaches a pre-specified level, the 3D-sequence is triggered.

• Centric-phase coding is used in conjunction with these techniques so that central k-space is acquired at the beginning of the scan when the vascular contrast is maximal.

Data processing

• A variety of reformatting techniques are now available. Each has its own strengths and weaknesses which can lead to pitfalls and artifacts in inexperienced hands.
• Subtraction of a pre-contrast data-set from the arterial-phase-data is widely using in 3D-gadolinium-enhanced MR angiography of the lower limbs to eliminate background noise and provide better visualization of small vessels.

Maximum-intensity projection (MIP)

(see Figure 4.5)

• This is the most common means of displaying data.
• The value of each pixel in the 2D-image is determined by the densest voxel within each row of the dataset. If a row contains bone or metal this will obscure any other detail such as the vessel lumen. To overcome this, MIPs are taken from different angles in order to fully evaluate a vessel.
• This method is well suited to a low background signal where arterial contrast is high. It relies on excellent vessel enhancement within the raw data.
• MIP renders a 2D-image of a volume of data, the thickness of which can be varied.
• MIP-images obtained from the entire data set are almost always con-taminated by wrap-around or edge artifacts. This can limit the visibility of vessels. Ways of eliminating overlying dense structures include reducing the thickness of the MIP, and editing-out bone. However, a thin MIP may not include the full vessel lumen and thus can over- or under-estimate vascular stenoses.
• A series of MIP-images can be generated which rotate through 180 degrees on 360 degrees.
• MIP-images are useful and are generally preferred by clinicians. However, the source images or thin-section reformatted images should be examined routinely because arterial dissection and non-occlusive thrombus can easily be missed on MIP-images.
• MIPs are very useful for determining vessel stenoses where there is little calcification but lack any sense of depth and are less suited for aneurysm morphology assessment.

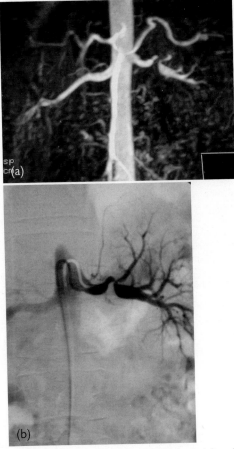

Figure 4.5 (a) Gadolinium enhanced MRA coronal MIP showing left renal artery stenosis and corresponding angiogram (b).

Volume rendering

- Volume rendering is now widely available on most new MR and CT workstations.
- Volume rendering displays voxels as virtual 3D-volumes, with objects selected by setting threshold values.
- Setting the threshold value is critical and data may be rendered non-visible if the incorrect threshold value is used.
- By varying the threshold, different tissues can be highlighted or hidden

- All the voxels contribute to the final image, being assigned different properties including colour, opacity, and brightness, depending on their attenuation values.
- By rotating the image, the 3D-anatomy is well displayed.

Reconstruction artifacts

Whenever the data is edited to produce a new image, information is lost. The resulting image may therefore be misleading. It is important to routinely review axial source images with the reconstructions.

Digital subtraction angiography (DSA)

- Now the standard way of producing angiographic images.
- Lower resolution than film-screen imaging but rapid acquisition and post-processing.
- Most units use a 1024-pixel matrix and allow switching between fluoroscopy and angiography simply and quickly.
- Images viewed either non-subtracted (raw) or subtracted.
- Acquisition up to 30 frames per second with continuous acquisition, used for bolus chase techniques and rotational angiography. Newer units can construct a 3-D model from rotational angiography data for complex embolization procedures.

Patient preparation

- Informed consent.
- Routine biochemical and haematology profile is checked (clotting profile on patients with liver impairment or anticoagulation).
- Patient monitoring with O_2 saturation, blood pressure, respiratory rate and heart rate are mandatory.
- The patient is positioned supine.
- All catheters and guide-wires are flushed with heparinized saline.

Technique

- Arterial access is gained, usually from the common femoral artery and an appropriate arterial sheath is passed over a standard guide-wire (see 📖 Chapter 5).
- A catheter, such as a 5F pigtail catheter, can be manipulated over a guidewire to a suitable position.
- The catheter is connected to a pump injector ensuring that no air bubbles are present in the system, or contrast may delivered by hand injection.
- Conventional contrast agent used is an iodine based non-ionic monomer i.e.:
  - iohexol (Omnipaque;™ GE Healthcare, Inc.)
  - iopamidol (Isovue;® Bracco Diagnostics, Inc.)
  - ioversol (Optiray,™ Tyco Healthcare and Mallinckrodt, Inc.)
  - iopromide (Ultravist;® Bayer Healthcare Pharmaceuticals, Inc.)
- Other contrast agents include carbon dioxide and gadolinium chelate.
- Selective angiograms of visceral arteries are performed using a variety of catheters and guidewires (see 📖 Chapter 3).

Acquisition of images

- Digital fluoroscopic images are acquired pre- (mask) and post contrast injection.
- Usually, up to four mask images are acquired prior to delivery of contrast.

Limitations

- Subtraction artifacts from involuntary movement, i.e bowel peristalsis or cardiac movement.
- Dose: Pulse fluoroscopy beneficial in reducing dose and preventing tube overheating.

Systems available

- Conventional Fluoroscopy systems (tube, table, image intensifier, video system) convert analog to digitized data using an analog-digital-converter (ADC).
- Digital video camera (charge-couples device) – resolution limited by the resolution of the camera to 1–2 line pairs/mm.
- Direct capture of x-rays with a flat-panel detector.

Image processing techniques

- **Last image hold**: last image hold uses digital information for the last frame and displays this on a reference monitor.
- **Grey-scale processing**: adjustment of the displayed contrast and brightness of the digital image (window width and level adjustment), allowing optimization of the anatomy of interest.
- **Temporal frame averaging**: decrease image noise by continuously averaging the current frame with one or more previous frames of digital fluoroscopic data. Increasing the frame averaging decreases the image noise.
- **Edge enhancement**: this increases the conspicuity of boundaries between objects of different pixel values.
- **Road Mapping**: following acquisition of a DSA sequence, the frame with maximum vessel opacification is used as a road-map mask. This is then subtracted from subsequent live fluoroscopy images to produce real-time subtracted fluoroscopy images. Used to guidewire manipulation during complex interventional procedures.
- **Mask Pixel Shift**: mis-registration artifacts occur when there is movement between acquisition of the pre-contrast and post-contrast images. It is possible to re-register the pre-and post-contrast images by shifting the subtraction mask with respect to the post-contrast image and re-subtracting the images.
- **Image Summation**: this is used to combine two or more frames of a DSA sequence into one image.
- **Vessel Size Measurement**: proper calibration of image pixel size using a reference object of known dimensions can be used to measure distances.
- **Bolus chase**: single contrast injection (70–80 Mls) to image entire peripheral vasculature using a stepping table or stepping gantry. Pre-contrast images are first acquired and subtracted from the post-contrast images. Timing of acquisition with the moving contrast bolus is critical and is operator dependant.

Maintaining good practice

- Always keep the C arm as close to the patient as possible (reduces radiation dose and artifact).
- Collimation to area of interest (better image and lower dose).
- Pulse fluoroscopy reduces dose. Low pulses perfectly adequate for catheter/wire exchange introduction. Higher rates or continuous or higher dose for critical stent deployments, etc.
- Use lead glass screens and undercouch lead protection. Keep hands out of primary beam and feet off the pedal unless there is reason to screen.
- Use previous imaging, i.e duplex, MR, previous angiograms, CTA, etc. to plan procedure and reduce runs.

Angiography using alternative contrast agents

Carbon dioxide, Gadolinium chelate

Alternative contrast agents to conventional iodinated contrast media may be required for arterial, venous, and non-vascular imaging in the following groups of patients:

- Patients with significant renal impairment.
- Patients with a known or suspected allergy to iodinated contrast media.
- Patients with a history of severe asthma.
- Diabetic patients taking metformin.

Carbon Dioxide (CO$_2$)

The physical properties of carbon dioxide which contribute to its suitability as a contrast agent include:
- Low atomic number and density compared with surrounding tissues gives negative contrast.
- High solubility (approximately 20 times more than oxygen), dissolves completely within 2–3 mins.
- Low viscosity and compressibility means CO$_2$ displaces and rises above blood. In a supine patient, with injection into the aorta, the anterior visceral arteries will fill preferentially. Makes it particularly sensitive in the detection of mesenteric bleeding.
- Low viscosity (400 times < iodinated contrast media) permits manual gas injection with small bore catheters with guidewires in place.
- Low viscosity permits improved visualization of collateral vessels in occlusive disease and after wedge hepatic injection.
- Naturally occurring byproduct of respiration so no risk of hypersensitivity reaction, hepatic, or renal toxicity. CO$_2$ is cleared by respiration.

Patient preparation
- Standard preparation for catheter angiography.
- No pre-medication with steroids or fluid bolus required.
- May be used for outpatient angiography.

Technique
- Conventional catheter placement under fluoroscopy.
- Patient monitoring with ECG, O$_2$ saturation, blood pressure, respiratory rate, and heart rate are mandatory to detect inadvertent delivery of excessive doses of CO$_2$ or air contamination.
- US Pharmacopeia grade CO$_2$ that is 99.99% pure should be used.
- Delivery by hand-held syringe (30–60 ml), a closed bag system, or a dedicated CO$_2$ injector.
- **For hand injection:**
  - Fill the syringe directly from the CO$_2$ cylinder via a sterile connection set.
  - Allow the syringe to fill without aspiration to reduce the risk of air contamination.
  - Connect directly to the catheter injection port and acquire images in the conventional way.
  - Wait 2–3 mins for complete absorption of the gas bubbles before subsequent injections.
- For closed-bag system:
  - Use a dedicated bag delivery system (AngioFlush III, AngioDynamics, Queensbury, NY).
  - The bag is filled with CO$_2$ and connected to the reservoir port on the AngioFlush III fluid management system.
  - This allows multiple injections and the airtight connections and valves prevent air contamination.
- Dedicated CO$_2$ injector:
  - A dedicated injector allows for reliable controlled delivery of CO$_2$.
  - It eliminates the possibility of air contamination or excessive delivery of CO$_2$.

- Studies show it reduces operator radiation exposure.
- It is expensive to purchase.
- Injection rate depends on the vessel's characteristics:
  - Aortogram : 30–50 mls
  - Mesenteric vessels 20–30 mls
  - Renal arteries 20–30 mls
  - Peripheral angiography: 20–30 mls with patient's legs raised to maximize distal vessel visualization.

TIPS AND TRICKS:

- Elevation of target vessel by 15–20 degrees maximizes distal vessel visualization.
- For renal angiography, tilting of the patient to the contra-lateral side maximizes filling of the ipsilateral vessel.
- Intra-arterial administration of 100–150 micrograms of GTN improves filling of distal vessels in the lower extremities.
- DSA with magnification over the area of interest improves visualization.

Contra-indications

Incorrect use of CO_2 may result in air contamination with the subsequent risk of air embolism. This occurs because air is much less soluble in blood than CO_2.

- Do not use in supra-diaphragmatic vessels because of the risk of intracerebral propagation and stroke.
- Exercise caution with patients with pulmonary insufficiency or pulmonary hypertension as it may increase pulmonary arterial pressures.
- Do not use in patients with right-to-left shunts, because of the possibility of paradoxical gas embolism.

Imaging in GI haemorrhage

In acute GI bleeds ensure:
- Patient has blood/fluid replacement available if not going in with a large IV access.
- Clotting factors checked.
- Plan of action discussed at senior level and patient if unable to embolize i.e. laparotomy or other.
- Has had endoscopy/colonoscopy as these will resolve the vast majority of cases.

Criteria for imaging in acute GI haemorrhage

- Evidence of active GI bleeding:
  - Haematemesis
  - Malena
  - Haematochezia
- Plus:
  - Haemodynamic instability (systolic BP <100mmHg, tachycardia >100 bpm).
- Endoscopy and or colonoscopy (all patients should undergo this before imaging).
- Radionuleide imaging.
- DSA.
- CTA (now most often the first line investigation).
- Capsular endoscopy.

Common causes include

- Ulcers (duodenal/stomach) usually treated by endoscopy.
- Malformations, i.e angiodysplasia.
- Diverticular disease.
- Meckels diverticulum.
- Tumour.
- Varices (usually treated by endoscopists).

Radionuclide imaging

- Uses either technetium-99m sulphur colloid or technetium-99m-labelled red blood cell (RBC).
- Radio-nucleotide imaging is non-invasive and is highly sensitive, and able to detect bleeding rates of 0.1–0.5 mls/min.
- Radio-nucleotide imaging is also non-invasive and is highly sensitive, and able to detect bleeding rates of 0.1–0.5 mls/min.
- However, its use is limited by the availability of both the isotope and gamma camera and is more often used in chronic bleeds. We will focus on the two main current techniques CTA and DSA.

CTA

- CT angiography is now established as the imaging modality of choice in the investigation of patients with acute GI bleeding, to establish the site and cause of bleeding prior to definitive treatment with embolization or surgery.
- Not all patients will require imaging;

- Endoscopy (+/−clipping/injection) is the primary investigation of these patients.
- Only patients in whom a diagnosis has not been established will require imaging.

Advantages

- Non-invasive.
- Readily available.
- May be repeated if initial imaging is negative.
- Animal models have depicted extravazation at bleeding rates as low as 0.3 ml/min with conventional single-slice helical CT.
- May establish the cause as well as the site of bleeding.
- Provides a guide for the interventional radiologist/surgeon prior to undergoing formal embolization.

Disadvantages

- Radiation dose.
- Possible additional contrast load.
- False positive results may occur if there is high density material within the bowel lumen such as iron tablets. This can be minimized by comparing with an unenhanced scan.
- The patient must be actively bleeding at the time of the examination in order to provide a positive scan.

Protocol for CTA in acute GI haemorrhage

- Suitable for patients in whom endoscopic examination had failed to identify the source of bleeding and who meet the above criteria.
- Phase 1:
  - 5 mm acquisition from diaphragm to symphysis pubis without oral contrast medium. Ensure the anal canal/lower rectum is imaged.
- Phase 2
  - 100 mls of iodinated contrast medium (Niopam 370) is administered by IV bolus injection via a 21G cannula sited in the antecubital fossa, at 4 ml/second.
  - Images are acquired in the arterial phase of enhancement centered on the abdominal aorta at the level of the diaphragmatic hiatus.
  - 0.625 mm acquisitions are reconstructed to 1.25 mm.
- Phase 3:
  - 5 mm acquisition from diaphragm to symphysis pubis at 90 seconds after the commencement of injection, giving a delayed venous phase of enhancement.

Diagnostic criteria for CTA in acute GI haemorrhage

(see Figures 4.6–4.7)
Positive study
- Luminal contents measure more than 100 HU.
- This is best assessed on the venous phase of enhancement as the addition delay allows for detection over longer periods.

- Arterial phase images are reconstructed to identify the vessel responsible for the bleeding.

Negative study
- A true negative scan may occur if bleeding has ceased spontaneously.
- The investigation may be repeated if there is further evidence of active GI haemorrhage.
- A false negative scans may occur where there is:
  - Artifact from metallic clips or implants (especially hip prostheses), or
  - High density material within the bowel lumen on the un-enhanced scan.

Venous phase images should be examined carefully in order to assess the bowel for a cause for intermittent bleeding, such as wall thickening, polyps or tumour.

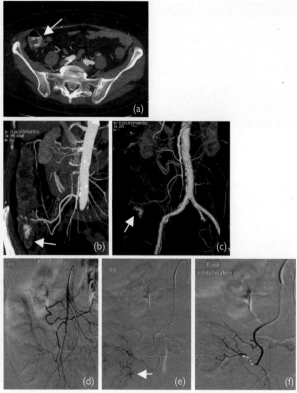

Figure 4.6 (a) Axial CT sections demonstrate active contrast extravasation in the caecum. (b) and (c) 3D reconstructions demonstrate branch of SMA supplying the caecum with a large draining rein suggestive of angiosysplasia. (d) and (e) IASDA confirms the site of haemorrhage (f), which was embolized.

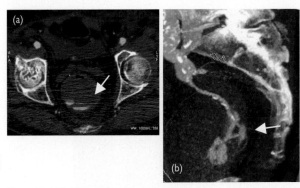

Figure 4.7 (a) Axial CT sections demonstrate pooling of contrast in the rectum. (b) Reconstructions demonstrate active extravasation from a branch of the arterior division of the right internal iliac artery.

Mesenteric angiography

(see also 📖 Hepatic angiography, pg. 191)

Advantages
- Gold standard (although CTA now taking over).
- Embolize at the same sitting.
- If unable to safely embolize then mark with methylene blue dyer or coil for surgeons.

Disadvantages
- Invasive and uncomfortable for patients.
- Small but real complications.
- Radiation.
- Large doses of contrast.
- Conventional digital subtraction catheter angiography (IADSA) requires the patient to be actively bleeding (greater than 0.5 ml-1 ml/minute) for a positive diagnosis.

Technique
- Aortography may be performed initially to demonstrate the positions of the mesenteric vessels (see below).
- Selective angiography of the coelic axis (Figure 4.8):
  - Performed using a sidewinder or cobra catheter with an end-hole and two side holes. The catheter tip should be positioned 2–5 cm along the celiac axis. The origin of the celiac axis originates anteriorly at T12/L1 level.
  - Pump injection of the coelic axis is performed using 25–35 mls of contrast at 5–8 mls/sec. Delayed acquisition of images during this run may provide portal vein opacification (indirect portogram), useful to confirm its patency.
- Selective angiography of the SMA (Figure 4.9):
  - Performed using a sidewinder or Cobra catheter with an end-hole and two side-holes. The catheter tip should be positioned 2–5 cm along the SMA. The origin of the SMA originates anteriorly at L1 level.
  - Pump injection of the SMA is perfomed using 25 mls of contrast at 5–7 mls per second. Again, an indirect portogram may be acquired.
  - It is important to assess for any anatomical variants (such as a replaced right hepatic artery), as these are common.
- Selective angiography of the IMA (Figure 10):
  - Performed using a sidewinder or Cobra catheter with an end-hole and two side-holes. The catheter tip should be postioned 1–2 cm along the IMA. The origin of the IMA originates anteriolaterally on the left at the level of L3.
  - Hand injection of the IMA is performed using 15 mls of contrast (at approximately 3 mls per second).

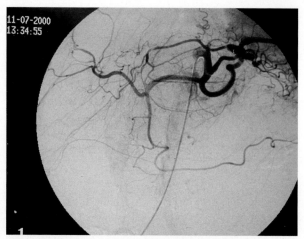

Figure 4.8 Selective celiac angiogram using a 5 F SOS Omni catheter showing classic hepatic and gastroduodenal anataomy with a unusually large left gastric artery.

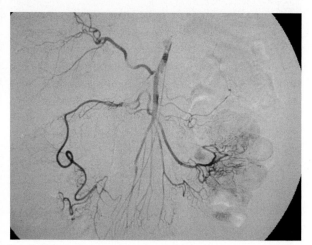

Figure 4.9 SMA angiogram using a 5F cobra catheter, demonstrating a replaced right hepatic artery coming off the SMA instead of the common hepatic artery.

TIPS AND TRICKS:

- **Knowledge of mesenteric anatomy is vital. There are a large number of anatomical variations which the operator should be familiar with, i.e. the common origin of the Celica/SMA, replaced right hepatic artery, origin of the the right and left gastric arteries, etc.**
- Oblique and lateral projections may be useful.
- Bowel peristalsis is common and causes movement artefact.
- Anti-spasmotics such as hyoscine butylbromisde (Buscopan) 20 mg–40 mg, repeated if necessary, are administered to reduce this.
- Provocation angiography may be performed. This involves the administration of heparin or rTPA directly into the mesenteric vessels prior to acquisition of runs in an attempt to recommence bleeding.

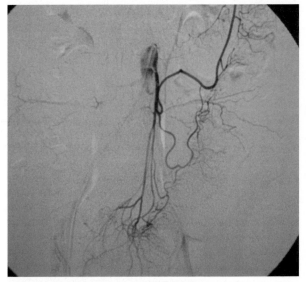

Figure 4.10 IMA angiogram using a 5F SOS omni catheter.

Assessment of angiograms for bleeding site

Look for
- Active extravasation.
- Spasm.
- Early venous filling.
- Abnormal tissue enhancement or vessels.

Arterial phase
- Extravasation, i.e puddles of persistent irregular contrast, not conforming to a vessel (Figure 4.11).
- Abnormal contours of vessels, i.e. aneurysm, strcture, displacement.
- Early venous enhancement (angiodysplasia characteristically has this). The ileocolic vein is normally the first vein to fill.

Capillary phase
- Abnormal capillary staining may be seen with angiodysplasia, tumor, or inflammation (Figure 4.12).
- Careful of overlapping bowel, and difference between small and large bowel. But may need obliques. Become familiar with normal enhancement appearances.

Venous phase
- Normal veins follow the same branching pattern as the corresponding arteries.
- Look for large, irregular or tortuous looking veins suggestive of tumor/malformation.

If the bleeding site is identified
- Try to embolize often using a microcatheters and coils. Particles/glue are more unpredictable (see 📖 Chapter 17).
- Vasopressin has been tried with mixed results.
- If not possible, inform surgeons, mark with a coil/methylene blue.

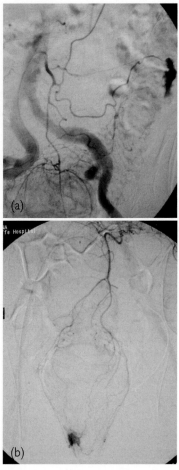

Figure 4.11 (a) Selective IMA angiogram using a 5F cobra catheter, demonstrating active extravasation of contrast from the ascending branch of the left colic artery, into the descending colon due to diverticular disease. (b) Active bleeding into the inferior rectum from a branch of the superior rectal artery.

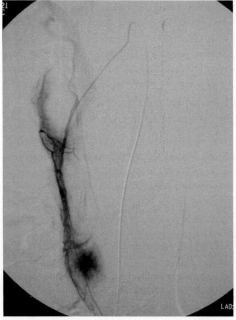

Figure 4.12 Selective angiogram of the right gastro-epiploiec artery showing abnormal capillary enhancement of the mucosa suspicious for tumor/malformation.

Mesenteric ischemia

- The history of this is key, i.e. thin patients who develop pain soon after eating.
- At least two of the three vessels will be diseased.
- The emphasis is on non invasive imaging, i.e. MRA or CTA, as described above.
- The techniques for DSA are similar to the above, but lesions are predominantly ostial, so prior to selective cannulation it is vital to obtain a lateral aortogram in order to look for origin stenosis.

Digital Subtraction Angiography in specific territories.

Pelvis and peripheral angiography

- If both legs are to be imaged simultaneously, then the legs must be positioned appropriately together and secured so as to intervene exposure.
- Retrograde puncture is performed and a pigtail catheter placed in the distal aorta.
- Contrast injection (non-ionic iodinated contrast medium), 370 mg iodine/ml, 30–40 mls at 15 mls/ second.
- Frame rate two frames per second.
- For images of the pelvic vessels, the patient is required to breath-hold during mask and image acquisition.
- The best breath-hold technique to use is in mid-inspiration or mid-expiration as extremes of the respiratory cycle have been shown to induce movement artifact due to abdominal musculature contraction.

Peripheral angiography

- If only one leg is to be examined, an antegrade common femoral artery puncture is performed (see 📖 Chapter 5).
- Dilute iodinated contrast (7 mls contast to 3 mls heparinized saline) is injected by hand through the access sheath.
- Standard projections include:
  - Femoral head downwards, often with ipsilateral anterior oblique angulation to intervene the origin of the superior femoral artery.
  - Femoral condyles upwards.
  - Top of patella downwards.
  - Ankle upwards.
  - Lateral view of the foot.

Aortography

Indications

- Evaluation of aneurysm prior to endovascular treatment.
- Assessment of atherosclerotic disease of mesenteric, renal, or pelvic vessels.
- Prior to selective angiography of visceral vessels.

Technique

- Via a common femoral artery access site, a 5F pig-tail catheter is positioned with the tip at the lower thoracic/upper abdominal aorta.
- Contrast injection (non-ionic iodinated contrast medium – see 📖 pg.14), 370 mg iodine/ml, 35–50 mls at 15–20 mls/ second.
- Frame rate two frames per second.
- A lateral projection may be useful to assess the origins of the celiac axis and SMA.
- For renal angiography 15–30 degrees posterior oblique projection may help to demostrate the origins.

Renal angiography

Indication
- Investigation of suspected renovascular disease.
- Investigation of renal tumours.
- Investigation and treatment of bleeding following trauma.
- Pre-operative assessment of a potential transplant donor.

Technique
Non-selective renal angiography
- Aortography is performed with the tip of the pigtail catheter just above the renal artery origins.
- AP and both oblique views are performed.
- Particular attention is given to identifying accessory renal arteries (25% of patients).

Selective renal angiography
- The tip of the selective catheter is positioned 1–2 cm into the renal artery. The renal arteries arise at the L1/L2 level, from the lateral aspect of the aorta, slightly posteriorly.
- Contrast injection (non-ionic iodinated contrast medium), 300 mg iodine/ml, 10–15 mls at 4–6 mls/ second (performed using hand intervention).
- Frame rate two frames per second.
- AP and both oblique projections are acquired.

Arch aortography

Indications
- Assessment of atherosclerotic disease of the carotid or vertebral arteries, inominate, or subclavian arteries.
- Evaluation of aneurysms and dissections of the thoracic arch prior to stent placement.

Technique
- Via a common femoral artery access site, a 100 cm long 5F pig-tail catheter is positioned with the tip in the ascending aorta, 5cm proximal to the origin of the innominate artery.
- Anomalous origin of the left common carotid artery from the innominate artery occurs in 25% of patients.
- Contrast injection (non-ionic iodinated contrast medium – see ⌑ pg.14), 370 mg iodine/ml, 45–50 mls at 20–25 mls/second.
- Frame rate two to three frames per second.
- 30–45 degree left posterior oblique views are used to evaluate the origins of the great vessels.

Trauma imaging

- This is now primarily imaged with CT which allows visualization of organ and vessels simultaneously (Figure 4.13).
- CT can accurately assess all the injured major organs, stage the extent of disease and guide operators as to which vessels to focus for intervention either surgical or endovascular embolization (Figure 4.14).

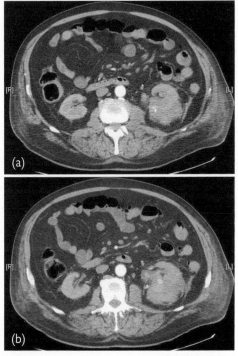

Figure 4.13 (a) Active extravasation of contrast into the kidney irregular renal margins consistent with renal capsular disruption and peri-penprhic haematoma. (b) Contrast is puddling in the collecting system.

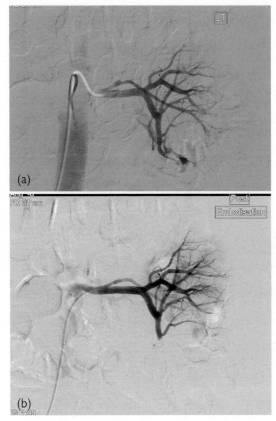

Figure 4.14 (a) Selective renal angiogram confirm AV fistula and a false aneurysm arising from a mid-polar artery. (b) Following successful embolization of the lower polar artery.

Further Reading

Anthony S., Milburn S., Uberoi R. (2007) Multi-detector CT: review of its use in acute GI haemorrhage. *Clin Radiat.* **62**: 938–49.

Kessel & Robertson. *Interventional Radiology – A Survival Guide.*

Arterial access for angiography and intervention

Patient preparation

- Nil by mouth for 2–3 hrs prior to the procedure, solids 6 hrs due to risks of aspiration following contrast and if sedation is required.
- Routine hematological and biochemical profile (including clotting screen in patients on anticoagulation or with known liver disease).
- Manage pre-existing drugs (see 📖 Medications pre-intervention, pg. 6).
- Informed consent is obtained (including discussion of non-serious but common complications and rare but serious complications).
- The patient is positioned supine on the angiographic table with both groin areas exposed and the skin is cleansed using 0.5–1% chlorhexidine solution.
- Sterile technique is used.
- The most commonly used site for puncture is the right common femoral artery (however, this may vary depending on the indication for intervention).

Access

It is always helpful to have an assistant.

Standard Seldinger technique

- Infiltrate 5–20mls of 1% lidocaine local anesthetic into the overlying skin and around the artery to be punctured.
- A small 5–10 mm incision is made in the skin and the soft tissue gently dissected with an arterial clip (i.e. Mosquito).
- The artery is punctured with a needle capable of taking a 0.35 or 0.38 guidewire (i.e. Sutton Potts, Seldinger, etc). If there is good pulsatile flow a guidewire is then introduced
- Guidewire; Either a straight or curved (J) standard 0.35 wire. J wires are less likely to dissect. 10–15 cm of wire are advanced into the artery and position confirmed with fluoroscopy.
- For diagnostic procedures a multi-sidehole catheter (i.e. pigtail) is introduced over the wire, with the assistant firmly fixing the wire out straight and 1–2 cm of catheter advanced , at the puncture site.
- For interventional procedures always use a sheath of appropriate size.

TIPS:

Wire won't advance

- Never use force. If there is resistance, screen the guidewire. A loop means possible dissection and the wire should be withdrawn and insertion re-attempted (Figure 5.4).
- The needle may be in the posterior or anterior wall, pushing the needle in or withdrawal may improve blood flow and allow wire passage. Contrast injection into the needles may be required in order to confirm luminal entry and exclude obstructing lesions. If there is plaque, changing the needle angle to redirect the wire may help (Figure 5.1). Try a different wire, Bentson is particularly useful (not-Terumo as the coating may shear off on the needle). If a dilator 4/5F can be exchanged then a hydrophilic wire can be used.
- Roadmap/Fluorofade may help.
- Re-puncture at a different site or alternative approach.

Catheter won't advance

- Make sure there is plenty of guidewire. May need a stiffer guidewire, i.e. Amplatz superstiff. Predilate with appropriate sized dilators. May need a sheath. Make sure there is no kink in the wire (more likely in obese patients). Use fluoroscopy. If there is then withdraw to straighten the wire and make sure the catheter is following the line of the wire as you advance.

Needles

These can be one part or two part. A single part needle only requires puncture of the anterior wall, and can result in subintimal entry of the guidewire if the bevel is not completely within the lumen.

Two part needles are simple to use but require a double wall puncture, i.e. both the front and back wall of the artery. This has a reduced risk of

dissection but has the disadvantage of potential hemorrhage from the posterior wall puncture, particularly for thrombolysis.
- Single wall puncture:
  - Thrombolysis
  - Lax surrounding soft tissues, i.e. arm, axilla, popliteal fosse or thigh.
- Double wall puncture (Femoral):
  - Trocar with shorter bevel
  - Easier to perform leading to fewer complications if operator relatively inexperienced.
- Wires through the needle: Either a straight or curved (J) standard 0.35 wire. J wires are less likely to dissect. Occasionally an Amplatz Stiff or Bentson wire. NOT Terumo as the coating can shear off the end of the needle into the artery and embolize.

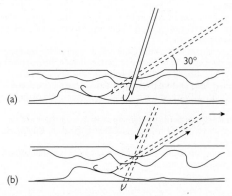

Figure 5.1 Correct angulation of the needle either with single puncture (a) or double puncture (b) technique i.e approx 30 degrees allows access to the largest area of lumen for introduction of guidewires. J wires less prone to dissect.

Access sites

Non invasive imaging, i.e. Duplex, MRA, or CTA is useful for identifying best access.

Retrograde femoral, radial, brachial, and subclavian approaches are used for diagnostic angiography or interventions above the inguinal ligament.

Antegrade femoral, popliteal, retrograde popliteal (sometimes used for iliac interventions as well) tibial vessel or dorsalis pedis approaches are used for infra-inguinal interventions.

Femoral

- Most commonly used for diagnostic and interventional procedures. Retrograde punctures are to access vessels above the inguinal ligament and antegrade for vessels below. Retrograde punctures are easier and should be the first technique to master before attempting antegrade punctures.
- The arterial puncture should be directly over the midpoint of the femoral head (Figures 5.2 and 5.3) in order to allow for good compression post procedure.
- Using landmarks such as the groin crease is unreliable resulting in high or low punctures. Fluoroscopy is used to identify the mid point of the femoral. Ultrasound can be invaluable in difficult punctures.
- For retrograde puncture (Figures 5.2 and 5.3) the skin incision is 1–2 cm below this (will vary with patient habitus) at an angle of up 30–45 degrees.
- For an antegrade puncture the skin incision is 23 cm above this
- (will vary with patient habitus) and at an angle of 45–60 degrees down (Figures 5.4 and 5.5).
- Never puncture above the inguinal ligament as it is impossible to compress the external iliac artery post procedure!

TIPS:

Antegrade puncture with repeated profunda femoris entry

If there is sufficient room between the point of puncture and the femoral bifurcation a curved catheter (i.e. cobra) can be used to direct the guidewire anteriorly into the superficial femoral artery (Figure 5.4). Another useful technique is to use a sheath with a side hole which is homemade or the sudeckny sheath (Cooks, UK) so that part of the sheath is down the profunda femoris and the side hole is directed onto the SFA to direct the guidewire (Figure 5.5).

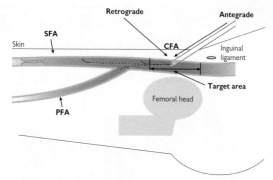

Figure 5.2 Lateral view of thigh. Target area (over femoral head) for either antegrade or retrograde puncture.

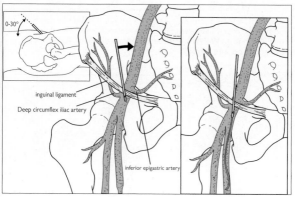

Figure 5.3 Antegrade puncture is the more difficult. Angling to 30 degree or less to the abdomen to puncture over the femoral head (below the inguinal ligament), prevents the needle directing the wire into the Profunda which faces posteriorly.

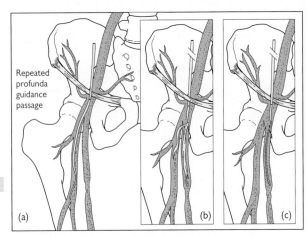

Figure 5.4 Use oblique screening i.e LAO for left side and RAO for right to visualize origin of SFA and curved catheter i.e. Cobra to enter SFA. (a) Catheter/wire in profunda. (b) Withdraw catheter into common femoral. (c) Use angled catheter to direct wire into SFA.

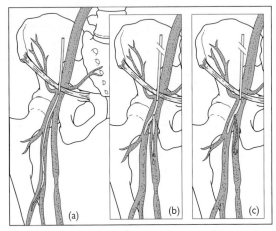

Figure 5.5 (a) Alternative technique for using catheter to get SFA access. If there is little room between the puncture site and SFA origin. (b) and (c) A catheter with large sideholes (Sudeckny) or sheath with a hole made in the dilator will allow the guidewire to be passed into the SFA.

Advantages
- Often shortest route to infra-inguinal intervention:
  - Greater control.
  - Clot aspiration.
  - Thrombolysis.
  - Easier stenting.

Disadvantages
- More difficult puncture:
  - Obese patients and previous groin surgery.
  - Hernias.
  - High lesion or bifurcation, i.e. distal common femoral/SFA origin.
  - Risk of high puncture or multiple punctures including inferior epigastric and circumflex iliac arteries or venous (AVM).
  - Low punctures with direct SFA/Profunda.

Puncture site complications
- Dissection-more likely with single puncture and inexperienced operator.
- Haematoma (0.2–4%):
  - Hypertension, Obesity, Catheter size, calcification, high heparin dose, Steroids, Collagen disorders, High puncture.
  - Reduced-CF puncture, Sheaths, > 10 min compression, low heparin dose and controlling blood pressure? Closure device.
- False Aneurysm – usually associated with haematoma (<0.5%).
- A-V Fistulae – More likely with double puncture technique and multiple punctures (<0.1%).
- Occlusion (<0.5%).
- Infection – Repeated use of same site/prolonged presence of sheath. Use prophylactic antibiotic when puncturing grafts.
- Femoral nerve damage Rare.
- Balloon impaction following rupture-less common with newer balloons which rupture longitudinally rather than circumferentially.

Difficult punctures

Obesity

You may require a longer needle and the skin incision will need to be further away from the intended puncture site of the common femoral artery directly over the midpoint of the femoral head.

TIPS:

A 16 gauge abbocath-T (Hospira, Donegal, Ireland) can be very useful and will allow access in all but the most obese patients for either a retrograde or antegrade puncture.

Tape the overhang of the abdomen up/laterally to the patient's chest or table to keep this out the way. An assistant could also do this.

Duplex ultrasound can be invaluable when dealing with deep or weak pulses in guiding needle puncture and should ideally be available in the interventional room at all times.

For difficult antegrade punctures, i.e. Obesity, hernia, surgical scars, colostomy/ileostomy sites, etc. the technique of retrograde to antegrade conversion can be invaluable.

(See Figures 5.8–5.10)
- Skin puncture 1–2 cm higher than the standard retrograde puncture.
- More vertical puncture, i.e. 60% to horizontal.
- Pass wire to aorta.
- Advance curved catheter, i.e. SOS, SIMMS 1, Shepherds crook, etc, (Figure 5.6),
- Pass soft wire, i.e. Bentson or curved Terumo.
- Bring wire back down into the ipsi-lateral iliac and then both withdrawn down into SFA until catheter just traversing puncture site (Figure 5.7).
- Advance catheter and wire down SFA (Figure 5.8).

Advantages
- Slightly faster.
- Fewer punctures.
- Reduction in haematomas.

Disadvantages
- Increased screening time.
- Higher radiation dose.

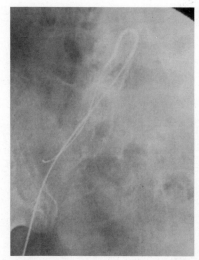

Figure 5.6 SOS Omni catheter with Terumo wire pulled into the common iliac artery.

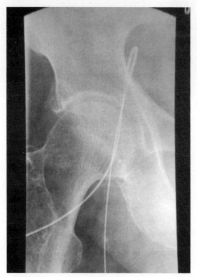

Figure 5.7 Now with guidewire directed into the SFA.

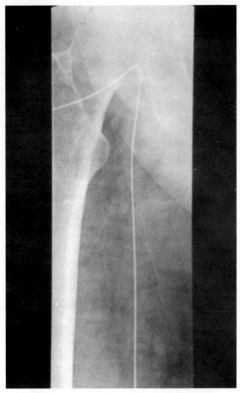

Figure 5.8 The catheter is then advanced into the SFA over the wire.

Other approaches, i.e. contralateral retrograde puncture with a crossed over the bifurcation sheath

Technique

- Perform standard retrograde puncture.
- Cross to contra-lateral iliac using pigtail or pre-shaped catheter, i.e. SOS, SIMMS, Renal Curve, Shepherds crook, etc. (Figure 5.9).
- Facilitated by Bentson wire, Terumo wire, Stiff Terumo and Super-stiff wires.
- Ipsi-lateral femoral compression to anchor the guidewire when catheter/sheath won't follow.
- A long sheath, i.e. Balkan, Arrowflex or Guiding catheter with a Tuhoy-Buhorst can be very useful when using the contralateral approach.

Advantages

- Simpler punctures require less skill.

Disadvantages

- Bifurcation can be very tight/tortuous, iliacs/severe disease resulting in failure.
- Less control even with contra-lateral sheath.
- Greater difficulty in dealing with complications.

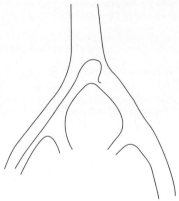

Figure 5.9 SOS Omni used to cross the bifurcation.

Alternative Access sites

Brachial approach

Useful when there is no femoral access or may be the first choice to treat subclavian, brachiocephalic, mesenteric or renal vessels. The sheath/catheter size is more limited in these smaller vessels. Cut down for larger sheaths, i.e. >7F.

The left side is preferred as it is often non dominant and crosses fewer cranial vessels.

Check radial and ulnar pulses before the procedure (perform Allen's test or use pulse Oximeter to look for desaturation during radial and ulnar compression).

Puncture from cubital fossa or above.

TIPS:

Duplex invaluable.

Use high brachial, i.e mid-humerus as the vessel is often larger and further away from the median nerve. The brachial artery is more mobile and fixing this with the index and middle fingers either side of it is helpful.

Duplex is useful in order to assess vessel size, duplication and guidance.

Use straight wires, i.e. Bentson to reduce likelihood of spasm. GTN/Nifedipine may be required if this occurs.

Curved catheters, i.e. Cobra, RDC, renal curve or even a pigtail are useful in directing the wire down the descending aorta.

Higher brachial punctures above the cubital fossa are less likely to cause complications.

There are complications in up to 8%.

The median nerve runs close to the artery and a major complication is nerve palsy usually due to compression by a large haematoma. Therefore careful compression post procedure is vital and avoid double wall punctures.

Radial artery access

Use a micropuncture kit. This is a used most commonly for diagnostic angiography and limited interventions particularly the renal arteries. It is important to assess the ulnar pulse first.

Advantages
- Superficial position makes it very easy to puncture.
- Lower bleeding complications compared to femoral approach.

Disadvantages
- Limited sheath size.
- Limited access for intervention to renal vessels and above.
- Failure rate of 4.8%
- Complications in 1.4% mainly arterial damage.

Axillary/Subclavian access

Useful if no infra-inguinal access. Elbow is flexed with the head resting on the palm of the hand. Artery is distal to the pectoralis major tendon fold.

The puncture is best performed with Duplex assistance. Larger sheath sizes can be used compared to brachial or radial approach and catheters/wires will easily reach the femoral arteries, depending on the patient's size. There is less catheter control than from a femoral approach.

Complications
Reported in up to 9.5%. Mainly neurological as the median and ulnar nerves are close to the artery.

Popliteal approach
(see Figure 5.10)

- 2–3 cm of reasonable above knee popliteal.
- Use Duplex guidance/Fluoro.
- Popliteal artery:
  - directly anterior to vein in 40%, anterolateral in 9%, antero-medial in 43%, other in 9%.
- Oblique medial angle to artery in the majority.
- Single puncture.
- Smart Needle may be helpful.
- Complications in 7.5% (Haematoma—4%, AV fistulae, etc.).

Advantages
- Lesions involving the Iliacs/common femoral artery or flush Occlusion of SFA when contra-lateral approach difficult.
- Potential to increase numbers suitable for treatment and successful outcomes.

Disadvantages
- Slightly higher complications.
- Limited sheath size.
- Limited ability to deal with complications.

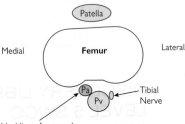

Figure 5.10 Axial view showing ideal line for popliteal puncture (PA & PV=popliteal artery & vein).

Retrograde Anterior tibial or DP puncture

Used as last resort to treat distal infra-geniculate or distal popliteal arteries when the antegrade approach has failed. This is used with the SAFARI technique.

A DP puncture is easier. Use a mirco-access kit using a 0.18 wire and 22 gauge needle. The artery can be punctured under fluoroscopy if there is already access from above, i.e. femoral, however it is usually straight forward with Duplex.

Venous DSA: This entails placing a 4–5F pigtail catheter into the right atrium from a femoral vein approach. Then 40–50 mls of contrast at 15–20 mls per second are injected and the arteries imaged on the delayed phase. Used primarily when femoral arteries are occluded. With other non-invasive techniques such as MR and CTA there is little need for this.

Venous Access

Prior non invasive imaging, i.e. Duplex, MRA or CTA is useful identifying best access. The technique is identical to the above. Important differences to remember

- Thinner wall vessels which will go into spasm easily (GTN, Nifedipine may help).
- Low flow so aspiration is required to confirm luminal position.
- Valsalva/Trendelenberg are very useful for distension of more central veins, i.e. Jugular, axillary, subclavian, femoral.
- Many superficial arm veins will already have been damaged.

Most superficial veins in the arms and legs can be punctured using a tourniquet and with contrast injection can help puncture more proximal veins.

TIPS:

Duplex is very useful in puncturing all veins (Figure 5.11).
Collaterals may be used, or the hepatic veins with Duplex/fluoroscopic guidance. Also consider direct IVC puncture or sharp recanalization of occluded vessels if there is a more proximal patent segment. 21 gauge needle and mircowire, i.e. 0.18 is usually required for initial puncture.

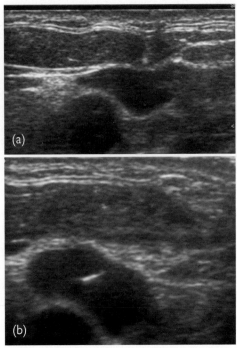

Figure 5.11 US guided jugular vein puncture. (a) Infiltration of the peri-jugular vein tissues with LA (b) Puncture into the jugular vein with a Seldinger needle prior to wire insertion.

Arterial thrombolysis and mechanical thrombectomy

Thrombo-aspiration

It is often possible in relatively acute thrombosis to aspirate a clot using a large sheath or guiding catheter. Aspiration is done using a guiding catheter, i.e. 5F for infra-popliteal or 6–8F for SFA and larger vessels (Figure 6.1). A Tuohy-Bohrst is placed on the end for haemostasis and the catheter advanced over a wire to the clot and aspirated using a 20 cm or > syringe. This works better with the wire removed. Sometimes the clot sticks at the end and the whole catheter has to be carefully retrieved from the sheath (a removable sheath is helpful here).

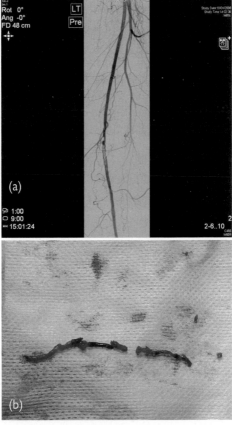

Figure 6.1 Aspiration using a guiding catheter.

Indication for arterial thrombolysis (AT) or mechanical thrombectomy (AMT)

- Acute onset of ischaemia in either a native artery or a surgical bypass graft.
  - This is usually a complication of an underlying stenosis, and therefore, the history is usually of an acute exacerbation of pre-existing symptoms.
  - Alternatively, acute arterial occlusion can occur due to embolization from a proximal source.

This distinction is not considered to be an important factor in making the decision to thrombolyze.

- Popliteal aneurysm, to try and open up run-off vessels for bypass grafting.
- AT and AMT are usually considered where the alternative option is surgery (surgical embolectomy or emergency bypass). The decision is based on the clinical and angiographic findings and the relative risks and benefits.
- A multicentre randomized trial (the Thrombolysis or Peripehral Arterial Surgery-TOPAS) found no significant difference between surgery and AT for acute limb ischaemia, with an amputation free survival at 12 months of 69.9% after surgery and 65% after AT
- Aspiration thromboemolectomy using a catheter with a large luminal diameter (e.g. 6F renal double curve guiding catheter, Cordis Endovascular, Miami, USA) and a removable hub sheath can be useful to reduce the thrombus load and to remove insoluble fragments prior to AT.

Contraindications to arterial thrombolysis

Absolute

- Recent surgery to the head, chest or abdomen.
- Recent haemorrhage.
- Recent significant trauma.
- Recent cerebrovascular event or intracranial neoplasm.
- Pregnancy.
- Coagulopathy.
- Within 4 weeks of grafting. Almost always an underlying surgical technical problem requiring complete revision.

Dead limb (complete muscle paralysis and sensory loss). It is vital that patients are appropriately assessed.

- Urgent surgery if limbs will not tolerate 12–24 hrs of lysis, i.e.
  - Poor capillary return.
  - Partial muscle paralysis and sensory loss.
- Lysis may be attempted if:
  - There is no muscle paralysis and no or only partial sensory loss.
  - Some capillary return and venous doppler.

Relative

- Suspected infection at the site of thrombosis.
- Multiple arterial or venous punctures.
- Severe hypertension.
- Age.
- Vein graft >3 days (vein irreversibly damaged) run off may be cleared for further graft.
- Knitted Dacron grafts. These rely on deposition of thrombus to become impermeable and lysis would make them porus and lead to extravasation.

Technique

- Non-invasive diagnostic imaging (Computed Tomographic or Magnetic Resonance angiography or duplex ultrasound) is useful to determine the location of the occlusion and to plan the approach.
- The arterial puncture should ideally be performed as close to the site of occlusion as possible but with sufficient room for access into the clear vessel (4–5 cm).

Options
- For CI:
  - Ipsilateral CF.
- For total Iliac:
  - Ipsilateral CF.
  - Rarely upper limb, i.e. Brachial or contralteral CF (take care to avoid clot falling into normal side).
- For External Iliac and CF:
  - Contralateral CF.
  - Rarely upper limb, i.e Brachial.
- For CF and below:
  - Contalateral CF.
- For SFA,Popliteal and run-off:
  - Antegrade CF.
  - Rarely contralateral CF.
- The ipsilateral common femoral artery is usually the access site of choice.
- If a diagnostic angiogram has been performed before the decision to commence thrombolysis is made, the same access site should be used whenever possible to avoid a second arterial puncture.
- A diagnostic catheter angiogram is performed, to delineate the anatomy.
- The occlusion is then crossed, usually with the aid of a hydrophilic guidewire. This should be achieved in the intraluminal plane whenever possible. Thrombolysis may be less effective if the occlusion is not crossed, but should be attempted if even a segment of the occlusion has been penetrated.
- A specialized thrombolysis infusion catheter is then passed into the occlusive thrombus (e.g. multi-sideport infusion catheter (Cook, Bloomington, USA, Figure 6.2 or multi-slit catheter (Angiodynamics, Queensbury, USA).
- The tip of the catheter is placed 1–2 cm within the occlusion, to allow a 'plug' of thrombus to minimize the risk of distal embolization and keep the drug in contact with the clot as long as possible.
- A tip-occluding guidewire is used, so that the thrombolytic agent is infused selectively through the side holes or slits directly into the thrombus.

TIPS:

A simple straight diagnostic 4F multisidehole catheter can be used if there is no specialist catheter.

For rapid lysis in long occlusions a combination of a long sheath and lysis catheter can be used. The sheath is placed into the proximal thrombus and the lysis catheter as distally as possible for simultaneous infusion of lytic agents.

Pulse spray is less commonly employed now but is rapid and requires repeated infusion of small aloquots of agent every few minutes, but requires the room to be tied up for 2–3 hours.

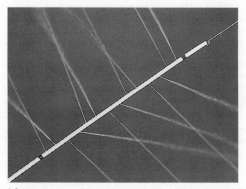

Figure 6.2 The multi-sideport infusion catheter (Cook, Bloomington, USA, reproduced with permission).

Thrombolytic agents

1. Streptokinase.
2. Urokinase.
3. Recombinant tissue plasminogen activator (rTPA).

There are two basic techniques for delivery of the thrombolytic agent.

Low-dose infusion thrombolysis

(see Figure 6.3)

- This technique employs a continuous infusion of a low-dose thrombolytic (e.g. rTPA 0.5 mg/hour. The patient is recalled for repeated angiography every 3–6 hours. The catheter is manipulated into an optimal position within the thrombus at these times, and the infusion is continued as long as there is an ongoing improvement in the angiographic appearances, usually up to a maximum of 36–48 hours. Thrombolysis is discontinued if the appearances do not improve in 12 hours.
- The patient requires intensive monitoring, ideally on a High Dependency Unit, during the infusion.
- There can be a clinical deterioration prior to improvement due to distal propogation of small emboli as the clot fragments. Thrombolysis should be continued during this time with an increased dose if necessary.

Accelerated thrombolysis

- The thrombus is initially laced with the thrombolytic agent, either by high dose bolusing (e.g. rTPA 5mg every 15 minutes to a maximum of 15 mg) or pulse spraying (0.66µg rTPA in 0.2 ml of water every 30 secs. The pulse spray technique requires a special injector.
- A high dose infusion is then commenced (e.g. 0.05 mg/kg rTPA/hour) for 1 to 2 hours. The procedure is discontinued at this time if there is no evidence of lysis. If there is evidence of improvement, a low-dose infusion can be commenced.
- AT, when successful, often unmasks an underlying stenosis, which can then be treated with either percutaneous transluminal angioplasty or stent placement.

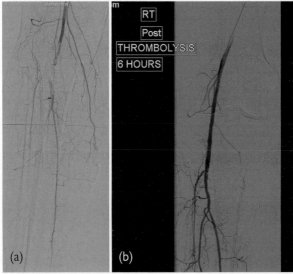

Figure 6.3 Acute thrombotic popliteal and peroneal artery occlusion. Pre (a) and post (b) thrombolysis.

Monitoring during infusion

- The patient requires intensive monitoring, ideally on a High Dependency Unit, during the infusion.
- A written protocol should be in place, which has been agreed by the Interventional Radiologists and Vascular Surgeons. The surgical team should be actively involved in managing the patient during the infusion.

Table 6.1: Monitoring protocol

Parameter	Frequency
a) Observations	
Pulse	Hourly
Blood pressure	Hourly
Puncture site(s)	Hourly
Temperature	Hourly
Urine output	Hourly
b) Hematology	
Full Blood Count	Daily
International Normalised Ratio (INR)	Daily
Activated Partial Thromboplastin Time	Daily
Thrombin Clotting Time	Daily
Fibrinogen	Daily
c) Biochemistry	
Urea & Electrolyes	Daily
Glucose (non-diabetic)	Daily
Glucose (non-insulin dependant)	4 hourly
Glucose (insulin dependant): with sliding scale	4 hourly

- Intravenous heparin at a therapeutic dose and warfarin are commenced after successful thrombolysis.
- The heparin is discontinued when the INR reaches therapeutic levels i.e >2.
- Warfarin is continued for 6 months.

Complications of arterial thrombolysis

- Major haemorrhage (7%): If there is evidence of significant haemorrhage, the infusion should be terminated.
- Initial clinical deterioration, with worsening rest pain: common. Requires adequate analgesia and continuation of treatment.
- Haemorrhagic or ischaemic stroke (1–3%): The infusion should be terminated, and appropriate imaging arranged.

- Puncture site haematoma (10%): may be managed by external compression. If unsuccessful, thrombolysis may need to be terminated.
- Distal embolization (10%): May be managed by re-directing the infusion, aspiration thrombectomy, or possibly surgical embolectomy.
- Allergic or hypersensitivity reactions: Extremely rare. Managed similarly to other allergies.
- Reperfusion injury, including compartment syndrome.
- Pericatheter thrombosis, as the catheters are left in situ for prolonged periods.

Percutaneous arterial mechanical thrombectomy

- AMT can be used either as a stand-alone procedure or in conjunction with AT for the treatment of acute arterial occlusions, either in native arteries or within surgical bypass grafts..
- Diagnostic imaging and arterial access are performed as for AT..
- A range of devices are available for use, and their mechanisms of function are summarized below, along with selected examples.

Hydrodynamic aspiration devices

These devices create a high-speed jet of saline at the catheter tip, which results in fragmentation and aspiration of the thrombus.

- The Angiojet (Possis Medical, Minneapolis, USA) is available in a variety of catheter sizes and designs, depending on the target vessel. High pressure saline jet(s) are directed back towards hole(s) adjacent to the catheter tip, resulting in fragmentation and aspiration of the thrombus.
- The Hydrolyser (Cordis Endovascular, Miami, USA – Figure 6.4) is also available in two sizes (6F Triple lumen device and 7F double lumen device). It generates a saline jet using a pump injector. The injection channel turns back on itself adjacent to the catheter tip, thereby directing the jet towards a side hole, through which the fragmented thrombus is aspirated.

Fragmentation devices

These devices mechanically fragment the thrombus.

- The Helix Clot Buster (ev3, Minneapolis, USA) utilizes a drive shaft, extending the length of the catheter, which rotates an encapsulated impeller housed at the distal end of the device. This creates a re-circulating vortex which fragments and disperses the thrombus.
- The Rotarex system (Straub Medical AG, Wang, Switzerland) has a catheter head consisting of two superimposed cylinders with side slits. The inner cylinder is fixed to the catheter shaft, the outer cylinder to a rotating spiral running through the whole length of the catheter and driven by an electric motor at 40,000–60,000 rpm (depending on the catheter type). The rotation produces negative pressure. Occlusion material is aspirated into the catheter slits, fragmented and transported to the outside by the spiral. No additional suction device is needed.

Ultrasound devices

Resolution (OmniSonics Medical Technologies, Wilmington, USA). This device has a flexible 75 cm long, 23-gauge applicator with a 5 cm long active distal tip (that potentially can be increased to at least 20 cm). The distal end of the wire has a 21-gauge ball that improves visualization and minimizes vascular trauma and the risk of perforation. A low-power transverse ultrasonic energy is generated through multiple, discreet nodes along the distal active portion of the applicator wire. This induces circumferential cavitation as far as 3–4 mm from the applicator, subsequently fragmenting the clot into minute, micron-sized particles.

Combined mechanical and AT devices

Trellis device (Bacchus USA) This is a device which utilizes two balloons 20 cm apart which have a multi-sideholed catheter in between and a rotational screw within this, so that when it is switched on between the inflated balloons it mixes the clot with the drug without distal embolization.

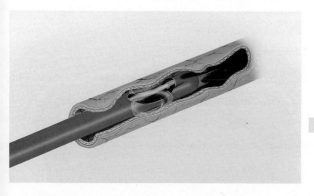

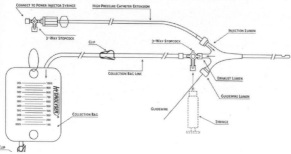

Figure 6.4 The Hydrolyser (Cordis Endovascular, Miami, USA, reproduced with permission).

Complications of arterial thrombectomy

- Distal embolization, either during manipulation of these relatively bulky catheter systems with in the arterial system or embolization of thrombus fragmented by the device.
- Vessel trauma: in theory, these devices are designed to avoid contact with the vessel wall, but mechanical trauma remains a possibility.
- Haemolysis and anaemia.

References

Earnshaw, J.J. (2004) Thrombolysis for acute leg iscaemia: 20 years and out? In: *Endovascular Intervention-Current Controversies*. Wyatt M.G. and Watkinson A.F. (eds). tfm Publishing, Shrewsbury, UK, pp 179–86.

Ouriel K., Veith F.J., Sasahara A.A. (1998) for the Thrombolysis or Peripehral Arterial Surgery (TOPAS) Investigators. A comparison of recombinant urokinase with vascular surgery as initial treatment for acute arterial occlusion of the legs. *N Engl J Med* **338**: 1105–11.

Müller-Hülsbeck S., Jahnke T. (2003) Peripheral arterial applications of percutaneous mechanical thrombectomy. *Tech. Vasc. Interv Radiol.* Mar; **6**(1): 22–34.

Angioplasty and stenting

Angioplasty

Indications

Pelvic and lower limb ischemia (short distance claudication, critical ischemia, blue toe syndrome) due to atherosclerosis or Takayasu's disease (TASC A and B). See Figures 7.14 and 7.15.

Contra-indictions

Related to any percutaneous intervention (Groin sepsis, bleeding diathesis or severe coagulopathy), TASC D.

Relative contra-indications

Anticoagulation, contrast allergy (CO_2 or Gadolinium as alternative contrast can be used), heavy concentric calcification of the aorta and TASC C.

Standard prepartion
- Check bloods, in particular electrolytes as administering nehprogenic contrast media.
- Aspirin commence at least 48 hrs before and lifelong if not contra-indicated.
- All patients have IV access.
- 5,000 units intra-arterial heparin in divided doses during procedure. More if procedure prolonged.
- Thrombolysis prior to procedure may be necessary in rare selective occlusions, particularly iliac arteries.
- Pre- post trans lesional pressures very useful in guiding therapy. <10 mmHg resting peak systolic gradient or mean of <5 mmHg = <30% stenosis and require no further treatment. Pressure measurements are very simple and can be performed with the external transducer connected directly to the catheter hub either as a pull back, or sequential through a sheath (to maintain wire position across a lesion or simultaneous with a second transducer/catheter.

Crossing lesions
- Plan the procedure well before.
- Have good imaging prior to the procedure. Use road map, fluoro- fade, reference images, rotational angiography, etc. to visualize where the lumen is and orientate the C arm to the tangential position in order to make life easy.

Stenosis

Equipment

- Always use a sheath. Protects access from damage from unfurled balloon, easier exchanges. Re-enforced sheaths useful in tortuous anatomy or when catheters turned from retrograde to antegrade.
- Curved catheter (cobra or multipurpose) and floppy guidewire (i.e. Bentson) or more commonly a hydrophilic wire. Curved wires give more direction.
- 5F systems give more torque control than 4F.
- Use torquers to direct the wire.

> **TIPS:**
>
> Wet Gauze swab, one way tap, or looping the end of the wire are cheap alternatives to pinvise torque devices.

- 3000–5000 units heparin is standard. Larger doses required for longer procedures, i.e. >1–2 hours.
- Give half as soon as access is gained prior to crossing.
- Obtain good quality images of the lesion with additional obliques if necessary to show path through stenosis.
- Gentle torque of the catheter and probing with the wire will allow easy crossing of the majority of stenosis (Figure 1a).
- The catheter directs the wire but with a curved hydrophilic wire also gives direction control and both may be needed to find the lumen. A Bentson is very soft and will buckle and flop through most stenosis, this and other wires need to be directed using the catheter.
- Advance 4–5 cm with the wire, then follow with the catheter and repeat until lesion crossed.
- Don't use force! If the wire buckles or loops it will dissect (unless using a Bentson) and you will need to perform a subintimal plasty and this is not usually necessary for stenosis. Also re-entry into the true lumen cannot be guaranteed. Subintimal may be used as a last resort in stenosis, however.

> **TIPS:**
>
> Struggling? Think of other approaches, i.e. popliteal, tibial, for SFA lesion, etc. Ask for help or come back another day.

Having crossed check position with contrast injection. Give rest of heparin. Exchange wire (may need stiff wire for extensive, tight lesions) tip is placed 4–5 cm distal to lesion.

TIPS:

In small vessels, i.e. below knee, arm, etc. use soft straight wires and pre-treat with anti-spasmodic, i.e. Nifedipine to prevent spasm.

- Never loose sight of tip of wire as this can damage distal vessels, particularly stiff wires.
- If catheter does not follow the wire, exchange for a still wire, use a 4 straight catheter, use a low profile balloon, i.e. 3 mm 0.18 system to predilate.

Occlusions

(see Figure 7.1a)

More challenging. Use same technique as above. Gently probe the occlusion with the wire, it may go on its own, may require a regular change in the direction of the wire and a curved catheter. The aim is to find the relatively soft more recently closed channel between the hard and often calcified plaque.

Subintimal: Advocated as the primary technique for occlusions by many and has potentially longer patency rates.

- Form a loop in the wire above or in the occlusion. Easier with a curved hydrophilic wire.
- Push with the loop (Figure 7.1b). Considerable force may occasionally be needed. Advance wire and catheter as above.
- The wire often re- enters below the occlusion at the site of collaterals. Be mindful of where they are and aim for them.
- When across the occlusion the wire will visibly jump forward. Check. Exchange wire.

TIPS:

If the loop suddenly widens, it has perforated. Check with contrast. Go back to the top and find another route.

If long hard, calcified lesion use a straight 4F catheter or tapered catheter, i.e. Van Andel.

Stiff hydrophilic wires may be used, but more likely to perforate, but may be useful to begin the sub-intimal tract and for catheter exchange.

For long occlusions, partial dilatation with 3–4 mm balloon of the proximal tract will allow passage of the catheter and balloon all the way across the occlusion/exchange for a stiffer wire.

If wire won't re-enter consider popliteal or even tibial approach.

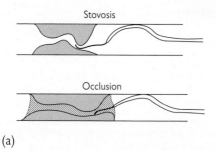

(a)

Figure 7.1a Occlusions.

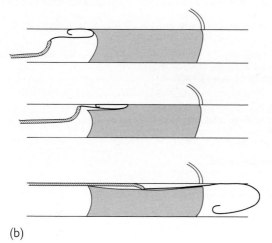

(b)

Figure 7.1b Pushing with the loop.

Dilatation

- Mark lesion position, i.e. clips on the drape or roadmap/fluorofade or reference image.
- Size the balloon diameter to adjacent normal vessel. See guide tables 7.1 and 7.2.
- Length goes from 1–16 cm. Treat only the diseased area in order to reduce damage. Longer balloons have less even radial force. Shaft length usually 75 cm for most lesions, but may need longer for different access or site, i.e. brachial/subclavian, etc.
- Use an inflator to get correct pressure. Most balloons are semi-compliant, i.e. will increase very slightly, i.e. fractions of a mm in size with increasing in pressure beyond 6 ATM.
- Burst pressure of balloons varies, decreasing with increasing diameter and size of balloon.
- Rated burst pressure means 99.9% of balloons will not burst below that pressure.
- Diluted contrast is used to inflate (30–50%) as full strength is too viscous and slows deflation dramatically.

Post Angiogram. Check not only treated sites but also the outflow and compare with pre dilatation imaging.
Residual stenosis, i.e. >30%.

- 1. Re-balloon up to three times.
- 2. Gently increase balloon size if the patient is comfortable.
- 3. Use high pressure balloon if waisting on standard balloon.
- 4. Return for cutting balloon in 4–6 weeks time
- 5. Or stent.

Complications

<5%.

Equipment related

Balloon rupture (Figure 7.2). Designed for longtitudinal tear and can be removed easily , circumfrential tear can ruck up and impact in the sheath and or shear/embolize distal end of balloon. Check balloon contour carefully on removal.
Catheter wire fracture: Rare, will require snaring and removal. See 📖 Chapter 21.
Vasospasm: Minimize by avoiding too much wire movement in small vessels.

- Glyceryl trinitrate 100–200 µg or verapamil 2.5 mg bolus directly into vessel.
- 'Quick inflation angioplasty of site of spasm.

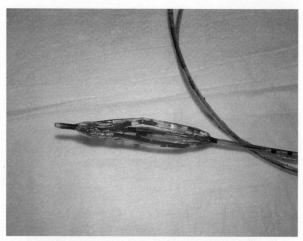

Figure 7.2 Balloon rupture.

Perforation/rupture: Wire or balloon rupture.

- Most will seal on their own or with simple balloon tamponade at 2–3 ATM. May need several 1 min. inflations.
- Superficial areas, i.e brachial, femoral. In addition to the above mark the site on the skin and press firmly.
- May require covered stentgraft, i.e. in iliacs (Figure 7.3).

Dissection: All angioplasties result in dissection.

- Flow limiting dissections may require gentle prolonged balloon tamponade.
- Stent if this fails.

Distal Embolization: If small in a minor collateral or unimportant branch vessel it may be appropriate to leave.

Significant emboli

- Thrombo-aspiration (see 📖 Chapter 6).
- Thrombolysis may be tried, but often there is an old clot or plaque which won't dissolve.
- Gentle angioplasty with low pressure balloon inflation.
- Stent if in a reasonable position.
- Surgery embolectomy.

Occlusion: May need a combination of all of the procedures above.

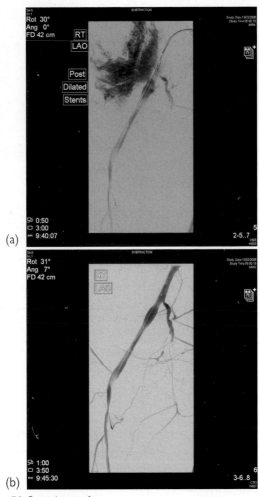

Figure 7.3 Covered stentgrafts.

Specific sites

Aorta
- Single balloon preferable (cutting balloon rarely used).
- Kissing balloons technique, if involving the common iliac origins and or distal aorta.
- Femoral access standard, bilateral for Kissing technique (Figures 7.4–7.5). Upper arm access for complex difficult lesion in addition.
- Size to < immediately normal vessel.

Patients (6-102)	Technical success	Clinical success	Primary Patency (years) 1/2/4/5/	Major Complications	Mortality
Range	83–100%	66–100%	90–100% / 80–89% / 70–93% / 64–70% /	0–18.5%	0–3%
Mean	96%	94%	85% (4–52 months mean follow up)	3.6 %	0.4%

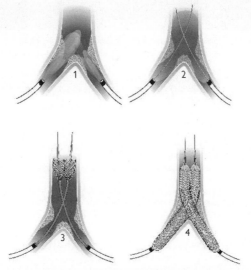

Figure 7.4 Steps 1-4 show the sequence of placing kissing stents to treat distal aortic/common iliac origin disease. The top ends of the stents are placed at the same level, approximately 15mm into the distal aorta, to avoid compromise of the either limb. © Cordis.

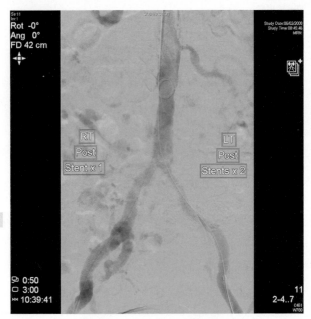

Figure 7.5 Completion angiogram following placement of kissing stents.

Iliacs

Approach as above, but also can use popliteal, subclavian/brachial and contralateral cross over approach.

- Stenosis often best approached initially by ipsilateral CF approach using a Cobra catheter and Terumo wire.
- Iliac occlusions even flush lesions are often more easily crossed by a contralateral CF approach although the ipsilateral approach should be tried first. A SOS or SIMS 2 are best for this.
- Form the required shape and pull snugly onto contralateral CI occlusion.
- Probe firmly with a Terumo wire with rotating motion with a torquer.
- Once across with guidewire try and advance catheter. May need a Van Andel or 4 straight.

TIPS:

- If the catheter won't follow and wire is being pulled back, try compressing the CF artery onto the wire to anchor it.
- Alternatively, try and pass the wire into the ipsilateral CF sheath, this is often possible with a 7F or larger sheath.
- Or use a snare to grab the wire and pull it out so there is a through and through wire (Figure 7.6) and a catheter can be then passed retrogradely across the occlusion. A wire can then be advance up to the aorta.
- Flush lesions may require kissing stents as above.
- If unable to get through from any approach the consider using outback catheter (Figure 7.7) which has a curved needle through which passes a 0.14 wire or alternatively use a contralateral balloon and ipsilateral refenestration using a Calapinto needle with the balloon as the target (Figure 7.8)

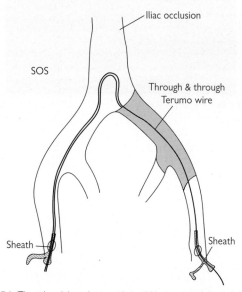

Figure 7.6 'Through and through wire technique'. Having crossed the occlusion using a curved reverse catheter i.e. SIMS 1 or SOS. The guidewire can often be advanced into the contralateral sheath. The sheath is gradually withdrawn and the wire pushed out with the sheath until the wire is out of the contralateral groin. More wire is pulled out and the sheath re-introduced with the dilator over the same guidewire. Alternatively, the wire can be snared and pulled out of the sheath.

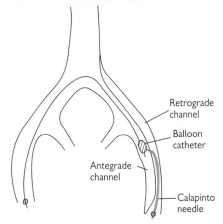

Figure 7.7 Re-entry catheter (Outback). © Cordis.

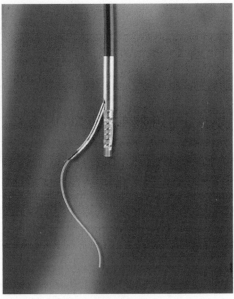

Retrograde
channel

Balloon
catheter

Antegrade
channel

Calapinto
needle

Figure 7.8 Having failed to break back into the true lumen, a balloon is introduced into the false lumen into the contralateral external iliac artery, and then targeted using a sheathed needle (e.g. Calapinto) to break from the true into the false lumen. The guidewire can then be snared and brought out of the ipsilateral sheath.

Common femoral
- Generally eccentric and calcified lesions and responds poorly to angioplasty. Works well for concentric lesions.
- Stenting contra-indicated across the hip joint.

SFA/Popliteal/Tibial vessels

Usual access femoral antegrade ipsilateral.

Alternatives
- Contralateral (particularly stenosis).
- Ipsilateral retrograde popliteal commonly used.
- Tibial retrograde as last resort.
- Stents being used more frequently (Figure 7.9). Higher risk of fracture than iliacs due to arterial mobility.
- Infrapopliteal.

Femoral antegrade
- Rarely tibial access if antegrade unsuccessful . Snare wire from the femoral access (SAFARI) and dilate as usual from balloon from above.

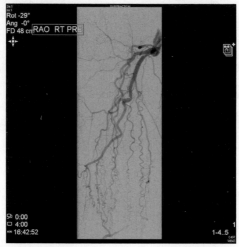

(a)

Figure 7.9a Use of stent in SFA vessels.

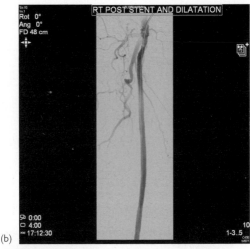

Figure 7.9b Post stent and dilatation.

Renal angioplasty

Indications: Uncontrolled hypertension despite maximal therapy. Renal failure.

- Size to normal vessel.
- FMH: Younger patients balloon angioplasty alone. May be bilateral and multiple.
- Atheroma. Older patients usually proximal, better outcome with stent (usually balloon mounted stent).
- Consider CO_2, contrast for angiography for patients in renal failure.
- Femoral or upper limb access.
- Equipment. 0.14, 0.18 and 0.35 systems available. Thinner wires allow for smaller shaft systems.
- Balloon angioplasty adequate for young patients with FMH, otherwise primary stent advisable.
- Most balloons require 6F sheath or 7F guiding catheter, i.e. Balkan sheath, Arrowflex or Hockey stick or cobra guiding catheters. These allow renal access, flushing and angiography during the procedure.

- Use Tuhoy-Bohrst to prevent leakage from guiding catheter.
- Cannulate renal areteries with SOS, SIMs or cobra catheter.
- Cross with hydrophilic wire, advance catheter beyond lesion. Exchange for stiffer wire and exchange for guiding catheter or curved sheath or may use balloon/stent wire (i.e. 0.18, V18 control wire).

- Dilate to desired size or pre-dilate prior to stenting (i.e. 3–4 mm to allow passage of stent).
- Check angiogram through sheath or guiding catheter. If poor angioplasty repeat balloon or consider stent.
- Stents may need further dilatation with larger balloons for inadequate result.

- *Important:* stents must protrude 2 mm into the aorta to prevent aortic plaque compression of ostia (Figure 7.10).
- Bilateral renals may be done at same sitting.
- Blood pressure may drop precipitedly, be prepared.

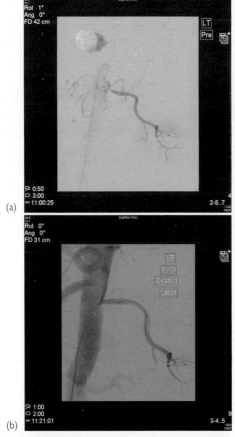

(a)

(b)

Figure 7.10 Renal angioplasty, pre-and post-dilated stent.

Celiac/mesenteric

Indications: Gut ischemia. Symptoms typically pain 30 minutes after meals. Patients usually thin.

Lesions
- Arcuate ligament web (celiac compressed as it passes through it). Usually not respond to angioplasty.
- Atheromatous stenosis.

- Use pre-imaging, i.e. MRA/CTA to plan case.
- Brachial/axillary or femoral approach
- Technique almost identical to renal stenting but worth attempting angioplasty first.

- From femoral approach, 6/7F sheath.
- Screen laterally and opacify the aorta with pigtail catheter to guide procedure.
- Cross lesion with 5F curved catheter, i.e. Cobra C2, SOS Omni or SIMs and hydrophilic wire.
- Exchange for tapered stiffer wire, i.e. Jindo or Amplatz stiff.
- 6F curved sheath or 7 F curved guiding catheter with a tuhy bohrst.
- Use short 2 cm 6–8 mm balloon. Size to adjacent vessels.
- Try three inflations for 20 seconds.
- If unsuccessful consider stenting. Use balloon expandable short renal stent (Figure 7.11).

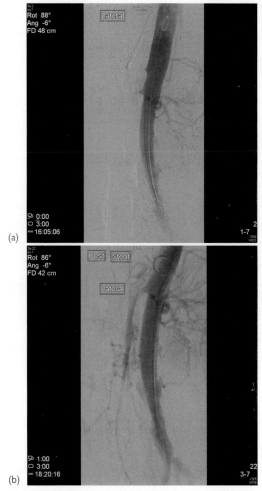

Figure 7.11 Balloon expandable short renal stent.

Brachiocephalic and subclavian artery intervention

Indications

- Upper limb ischemia (arm claudication).
- Vertebral steal (dizziness fainting particularly during manual labour).

Equipment: as above but also arch selective catheters (see 📖 Chapter 3) and long guiding catheters or sheath (6–8F).

Access

- Femoral (larger vessel if stenting) familiar access. Brachial (shorter route and greater catheter/wire torque). Vessel needs to be >4 mm particularly if large sheaths are required i.e. For stenting.

Technique

(see Figure 7.12)

- Similar to above, need arch angiogram to confirm anatomy.
- Advance guiding catheter to arch.
- Use selective catheter to access vessel, i.e. headhunter, vertebral, etc.
- Cross lesion with hydrophilic wire.
- Advance catheter and exchange for 180/260 stiff wire, i.e. Amplatz
- Advance guiding catheter to or just into origin.
- Angioplasty and or stent with completion angiogram through guiding cantheter.

TIPS:

If there is retrograde flow in the vertebral prior to the procedure this takes several minutes to go back to antegrade.
Avoid ballooning or stenting across vertebral artery if patent.

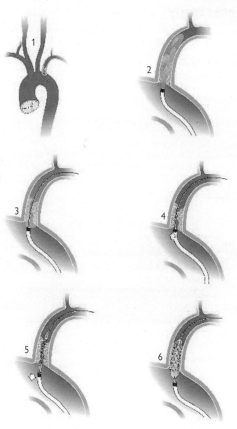

Figure 7.12 Brachiocephalic and subclavian artery intervention technique.

Atherectomy

Unlike angioplasty this cuts out atheroma. Silver Hawk is the only current device (Figure 7.13). There are different sizes for SFA/POP or run off vessels.

- 6F sheath or larger depending on device.
- Cross lesion in usual way.
- Exchange for a 0.14 wire.
- Need to pass across lesion several times cut in different planes, i.e. 12 o'clock, 3 o'clock in four quadrants.
- When cutting chamber is full the device removed and plaque flushed out of the chamber.
- Re-angiogram and repeat as necessary.
- Do not rotate 360 degrees or more in one direction as the wire will get caught. Rotate one way then the opposite way up to 270 degrees.

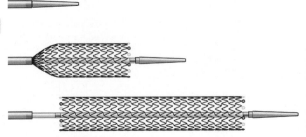

Figure 7.13 Silver Hawk. © Cordis.

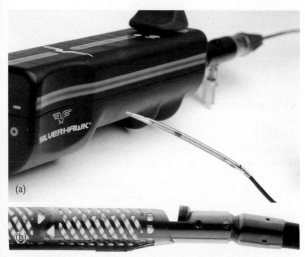

Figure 7.13a & b Silver Hawk.

Bare stents

Indications

- *Primary stenting* (without previous angioplasty).
- *Iliac arteries:* Some data to suggest better long term patency than balloon angioplasty alone particularly long occlusions.
- Patency > in stenosis than occlusions, shorter lesions, common iliac better than external and good run off vessels.

Secondary stenting following angioplasty

- Flow limiting dissection.
- Residual resting gradient across lesion >10 mmHg.
- Also consider in recurrent stenosis.

Femoral artery

Primary stenting

Data less clear for primary stenting. Some suggestion of longer patency with the newer Nitinol stents and drug eluting stents.

Secondary stenting

- Poor result following PTA.
- Flow limiting dissection.
- Also consider in recurrent stenosis.

Technique

Balloon mounted

- Usually short 1–6 cm (Palmaz-Cordis). Good for accurate placement, i.e flush lesions at the iliac bifurcation. Have the strongest radial force and maintain a better lumen when performing kissing stents in the iliac arteries.
- Most now pre-crimped on a balloon, but some still require self crimping by hand. Valve busters prevent dislodgement during placement through sheath.

TIPS:

The cut portion of the sheath the same size works just as well as a valve buster to allow safe passage of the stent on the balloon.
Not good for tortuous arteries.
Long sheaths advisable to reduce risk of dislodgement during placement.

Self expanding

- Better for tortuous arteries.
- Several types from the old Wall stent to the newer multiple varieties of Nitinol stents including the drug eluting and carbon coated stents. Also very new resorbable stents.
- Some data suggests longer patency with the Nitinol stents in the femoral arteries.
- Generally delivery systems consist of an outer sleeve which contrains the stent on the deployment shaft and there are different mechanisms to pull the sheath back and expose the stent distal to proximal (Figure 7.14). Markers usually present on the stents and sheath.
- The Wall stents are great stents but unlike the Nitinol stents which don't shorten during deployment, these can shorten up to 40%. Therefore not good for accurate placement.

TIPS:

Kissing stents useful to treat distal aortic or unilateral or bilateral common iliac origin disease (Figures 7.4–7.5).
Place both stents at exactly the same height approximately 15 mm into the distal aorta.
Balloon expandable stents have a greater radial force and more concentric and even lumen than self expanding stents.
Not advisable to treat lesions which show marked residual waisting during angioplasty.

TASC classification

Type A lesions

- Unilateral or bilateral stenoses of CIA
- Unilateral or bilateral single short
  (≤3 cm) Stenosis of EIA

Type B lesions:

- Short (≤3 cm) stenosis of infrarenal aorta
- Unilateral CIA occlusion
- Single or multiple stenosis totaling 3–10 cm
  involving the EIA not extending into the CFA
- Unilateral EIA occlusion not involving the origins of
  internal iliac or CFA

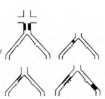

Type C lesions

- Bilateral CIA occlusions
- Bilateral EIA stenoses 3–10 cm long not extending
  into the CFA
- Unilateral EIA stenosis extending into the CFA
- Unilateral EIA occlusion that involves the origins of
  internal iliac and/or CFA
- Heavily calcified unilateral EIA occlusion with or
  without involvement of origins of internal iliac and/or CFA

Type D lesions

- Infra-renal aortoiliac occlusion
- Diffuse disease involving the aorta and both iliac
  arteries requiring treatment
- Diffuse multiple stenoses involving the unilateral CIA,
  EIA, and CFA
- Unilateral occlusion of both CIA and EIA
- Bilateral occlusions of EIA
- Iliac stenoses in patients with AAA requiring treatment
  and not amenable to endograft placement or other
  lesions requiring open aortic or iliac surgery

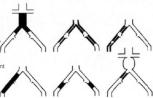

Figure 7.14 TASC classification of aorto-iliac lesions. From Norgren L, Hiatt WR, Dormandy JA et al; TASC II Working Group. (2007). Inter-Society Consensus for the Management of Peripheral Arterial Disease (TASC II). Available at: www.tasc-2-pad.org. Accessed 8th April 2008. Also published in *Eur J Endovasc Surg.* 33(Suppl 1): S1-75, *J Vasc Surg.* 45(Suppl S): S5-67 and *Int Angiol* **26**(2): 81–157. Reproduced with permission.

Type A lesions

- Single stenosis ≤10 cm in length
- Single occlusion ≤5 cm in length

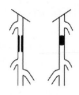

Type B lesions:

- Multiple lesions (stenoses or occlusions),
  each ≤5 cm
- Single stenosis or occlusion ≤15 cm not
  involving the infra geniculate popliteal artery
- Single or multiple lesions in the absence
  of continuous tibial vessels to improve
  inflow for a distal bypass
- Heavily calcified occlusion ≤5 cm in length
- Single popliteal stenosis

Type C lesions

- Multiple stenoses or occlusions totaling
  >15 cm with or without heavy calcification
- Recurrent stenoses or occlusions that need
  treatment after two endovascular interventions

Type D lesions

- Chronic total occlusions of CFA or SFA
  (>20 cm, involving the popliteal artery)
- Chronic total occlusion of popliteal artery
  and proximal trifurcation vessels

Figure 7.15 TASC classification of femoral popliteal lesions. From Norgren L, Hiatt WR, Dormandy JA et al; TASC II Working Group. (2007). Inter-Society Consensus for the Management of Peripheral Arterial Disease (TASC II). Available at: www.tasc-2-pad.org. Accessed 8th April 2008. Also published in *Eur J Endovasc Surg.* 33(Suppl 1): S1-75, *J Vasc Surg.* 45(Suppl S): S5-67 and *Int Angiol* **26**(2): 81–157. Reproduced with permission.

Table 7.1 Common balloon size for vessels. Lower limb

Vessel	Male	Female
Abdominal aorta	14–18	12–16
Celiac	6–8	6–8
SMA	6–8	6–8
Common Iliac	8–10	7–9
External Iliac	7–8	6–8
Common Femoral	6–7	6–7
Superficial Femoral	5–7	4–7
Popliteal artery	4–6	4–6
Tibioperoneal trunk	3–4	3–4
Crural vessels	2–3	2–3

Table 7.2 Common balloon size for vessels. Upper limb

Vessel	Male	Female
Thoracic aorta	18–24	18–24
Carotid artery	5–7	5–7
Brachiocephalic artery	7–9	7–9
Subclavian	6–8	6–8
Axillary	6–7	6–7
Brachial	5–6	5–6
Radial/Ulnar	3–4	3–4

Carotid interventions

Introduction

Of all the endovascular interventions, carotid artery stenting (CAS) remains the procedure with the steepest learning curve and the lowest margin for error. The procedure demands a meticulous approach, advanced catheter and guidewire skills, an excellent appreciation of neuroanatomy and the ability to manage dynamic fluctuations in haemodynamic status. Of equal importance is the decision-making and judgment necessary for appropriate patient selection.

This chapter will focus entirely on the technical aspects of CAS. It will be assumed that the decision to intervene on a significant carotid stenosis, whether or not it has given rise to neurological symptoms, has been a sound one. For the protection of both the patient and the interventionist, decision making within the remit of a multidisciplinary team attended by stroke physicians or neurologists with an interest in stroke prevention is advisable (NICE guidance IPG191) (1).

Access

- Extremely important aspect of the procedure.
- *Sustained* access to the common carotid artery (CCA) adjacent to lesion is vital.
- Avoid situations where long-sheath/guiding catheter is unstable and 'backs off' leaving, a untreated lesion and fully deployed protection device in the distal internal carotid artery (ICA) on a relatively non-supporting 0.014 guidewire.
- Difficult access is the commonest cause of a prolonged procedure (i.e. lasting more than one hour). May result in repeated catheter/guidewire movements and contrast injections increasing the risk of cerebrovascular embolic complications.

For more detailed review/discussion see Further Reading (2).

There are three main techniques for CCA access: the 'exchange technique', the 'co-axial' or telescoping technique, and direct probing. The access manoeuvre utilized is to some extent specialty-specific – a number of 'species' perform carotid stenting to include interventional radiologists, neurointerventional radiologists, interventional cardiologists, interventional neurologists, vascular surgeons and angiologists. Interventional cardiologists are more comfortable with the 'direct probing' technique, i.e. engagement of the CCA origin with a pre-shaped 8F guiding catheter. The 'exchange technique', however, is routinely employed to teach novices because of the (generally) secure and stable access that it provides.

Standard exchange technique

- Arterial access: See 📖 Chapter 5.
- Ultrasound-guided access is useful because it is highly likely that a closure device will be utilized at completion and ultrasound allows evaluation of the status and calibre of the access artery.
- The common femoral artery (CFA) is the most frequently used point of access for carotid artery stenting, although brachial, radial, and CCA access have all been described.

- A 6F short sheath is placed via the CFA.
- The patient is Heparinized at arterial access; 5,000–7,000 units are given (depending on the patient's size/weight and/or Activated Partial Thromboplastin Time. It is the duty of one of the nurses involved in the procedure to document the time of administration of the Heparin. A further aliquot of 2,000 units may be given if the procedure is prolonged. Appropriate selection of the patient based on anatomic criteria assessed on pre-procedure 'overview' imaging (3) should ensure that prolonged procedures are less likely.
- The catheter appropriate to the CCA to be catheterized is chosen.
- For 'straightforward' arches, i.e. 'Type 1' (Figure 7.16) (4), a 100cm 5F headhunter is adequate for most brachiocephalic and right CCA engagements and a 100cm 5F vertebral for the left CCA.

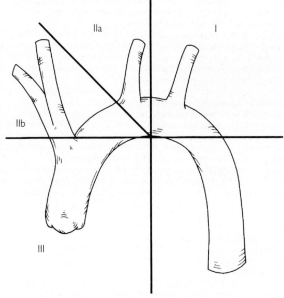

Figure 7.16 Different arch origins for the carotid arteries I-III which require different catheter approaches and increasing complexity.

- For Types II and III arches and a conjoint brachiocephalic/left CCA origin (i.e. a 'bovine-type' arch) recurrent curve catheters such as the sidewinder 2 or 3, Mani or Vitek catheters may be more appropriate, preferably 6F to ensure improved one-to-one torque.
- Once the CCA has been catheterized, the radiographer is instructed to position the image intensifier in the appropriate oblique projection to open out the carotid bifurcation so that there is no overlap between the origin of the external carotid artery (ECA) and the ICA. This projection can be chosen in advance by recourse to prior 'overview' imaging, i.e. from arch origin to circle of Willis, be that by CTA, MRA or catheter arch aortography.
- Ten millimetres of full strength non-ionic monomeric iodinated contrast such as iohexol (240 mg iodine/ml) is appropriate for selective injections.
- The ECA is selectively catheterized on road-mapping after instructing the patient to stop swallowing (which is best achieved after allowing several prior swallows), to close their eyes so that blinking does not interfere with the road map and to keep still.
- The straightest most respectable-looking branch of the ECA (most commonly the posterior occipital or the superficial temporal) is targeted. These branches allow the longest, most secure access route. A hydrophilic steerable 0.035 guidewire (e.g. Terumo) is advanced into the chosen branch under road-mapping.
- The selective catheter is advanced over the hydrophilic guidewire and the latter subsequently exchanged for a 300 cm exchange-length 0.035 guidewire with serious 'support' characteristics such as the Amplatz Superstiff (Cook Inc, Bloomington, Illinois USA). The hydrophilic guidewire should be removed in a moderately slow, steady fashion to avoid entraining air into the catheter on its removal. Although the catheter tip is in an ECA branch, some individuals have sizeable ECA to ICA collaterals and any air introduced into the ECA can thus end up in the ICA territory. The 1 cm floppy tip version of the Amplatz Superstiff provides substantial support throughout almost all of its length, but of course, caution must be exercised with its tip, which is unforgiving.
- In order to advance the stiff guidewire out of the end of the catheter in the chosen ECA branch, the catheter is usually pulled back slightly to allow the guidewire to advance (this is a two-handed manoeuvre).
- The scrubbed assistant may help to remove the catheter over the stiff guidewire whilst the first operator employs fluoroscopy and supports the short 6F sheath.
- The short 6F sheath is removed and a long 6F Sheath (such as the Introducer Guide, Cordis, Johnson & Johnson, Warren, New Jersey) is advanced over the Superstiff guidewire. This long sheath has an 8F-equivalent outer diameter. Alternatively, an 8F pre-shaped guiding catheter can be used.
- The end of the long sheath (with radiopaque marker) is positioned some 2 cm caudal to the carotid bifurcation lesion and the dilator and stiff guidewire removed.

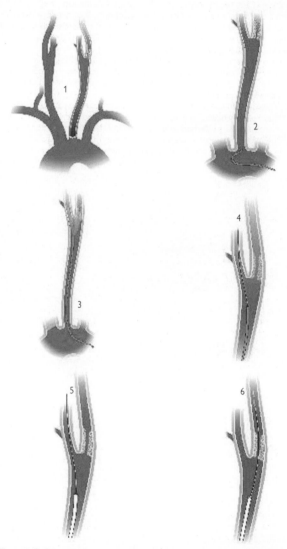

Figure 7.17 Schematic representation 1-6 of the first part of the procedure from cannulation of the left common carotid artery through to crossing the stenotic lesion. © Cordis.

If there is any recurrency/tortuosity of the CCA, the long sheath will fall around 1–2 cm on removal of the stiff guidewire. It is therefore useful to have a relatively high starting position, to allow for this, after all, it is relatively easy to subsequently pull the long sheath back slightly in order to deploy the trailing end of the carotid stent.

- Now the long sheath is securely in place. The sheath has a relatively large dead-space so this must be aspirated via the side-arm and around 5 mls or so of blood and air from the two-way tap on the end of the side-arm discarded.
- A pressurized bag of heparinized saline (set above the patient's systolic blood pressure), having been prepared beforehand and scrutinized for microbubbles, is attached to the side-arm of the sheath and continuous flushing of the sheath is therefore ensured throughout the procedure, in order to discourage the formation of thrombus within it.

TIPS AND CAUTIONARY TALES:

- Always ensure a fluid-to-fluid interface when injecting into the carotid arteries. The barrel of the 10 mm leuer -lock syringe should be held at a 45 degree angle and the barrel tapped to encourage any air to reside in the uppermost part of the barrel.
- The full volume contained in the syringe should not be injected – the last few millimetres will contain air.
- Blood/contrast mixes within syringes should not be injected into the carotid circulation. Microthrombi may be inadvertently injected. These may be irrelevant when dealing with an aortic aneurysm or infrainguinal angioplasty but suddenly assume much greater relevance when the end organ is the brain.
- The patient should be warned that in addition to a sensation of warmth, facial, perineal and otherwise, and of voiding, that they may 'see' sparkling lights, lightning, etc. as the viscous contrast agent circulates through the retinal circulation. Some may feel as if their mouths have filled with fluid. Forewarned is forearmed. These patients should not be sedated – their compliance is vital and they must be reassured in advance that most of what they feel during CAS is normal and to be expected.
- The lingual branch of the ECA should be avoided for the exchange technique. If the tip of the superstiff wire (Amplatz or otherwise), perforates this branch, there may be life-threatening airway compromise due to bleeding into the base of the tongue.
- When the superstiff guidewire is advanced into the chosen ECA branch, the patient may feel discomfort behind the ear or wherever is relevant to the branch chosen. The branch is likely to go into spasm but this is largely without clinical sequelae.
- For recurrent great vessel origins or tortuous CCAs, the patient can be invaluable in assisting the tracking of catheters over guidewires by either deep inspiration (to alter the CCA approach) or head/neck rotation.
- For bovine-type arches (particularly type III bovine arches – a configuration to be avoided at all costs whilst on the steep and slippery portion of the learning curve), a 6F sidewinder III catheter and a long-floppy tip, i.e. (6 cm floppy tip) hydrophilic guidewire can prove to be a winning combination and will at least allow engagement of the CCA origin.

Calibrated angiography

- Accurate sizing of the protection device and stent is mandatory during carotid stenting. The intimal lining of the distal ICA is perilously thin and provoking it with an oversized stent or protection device is asking for trouble.
- The stent is chosen by measuring the size of the CCA just below the bifurcation. The distal protection device (CPD), most commonly of filter-type (75% of current CAS episodes) is sized against the distal ICA.
- Calibration for accurate sizing of the stent may be performed on ultrasound prior to the CAS procedure. The distal ICA may be measured, giving the appropriate size parameters of the protection device to be selected but, of course, sometimes the distal ICA is not well demonstrated on ultrasound.
- The most important aspect of 'calibration' be that by ultrasound, catheter angiography in orthogonal projections relying on a two-pence piece of known dimensions (26 mm) or on calibration tools inherent in the angiography equipment is that the operator is convinced of or has been assured of its reliability (Figure 7.18).
- Once calibrated angiography has been performed, the most appropriate sizes of stent and filter are chosen. These are then prepared so that the procedure runs seamlessly once the lesion has been crossed.
- The stent is typically oversized by around 1–2 mm relative to the CCA diameter below the bifurcation. The degree of oversizing that is appropriate varies depending on the stent used. The cobalt-chromium Wallstent (Boston Scientific, Natick, Massachusetts) has relatively low radial force and may be oversized more than, for example, the Nitinol Precise (Cordis, Johnson and Johnson, Warren, New Jersey), which has substantial radial force. Inappropriately enthusiastic oversizing of stents with high radial force will result in more profound derangements of blood pressure and may risk dissection of the ICA.

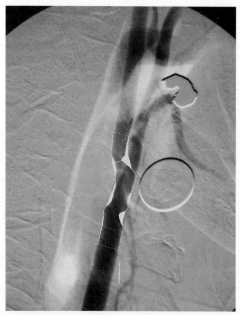

Figure 7.18 Calibrated angiogram using a coin of known dimensions. The software is calculating the precise dimension of the vessels and is able to calculate the percentage stenosis as by NASCET and or ECST crtieria.

TIPS:

To calibrate against a two-pence piece, the coin is placed over the carotid bifurcation in the frontal projection – small injections of contrast assist the radiographer in accurate coin placement. The coin is stuck onto the patient's skin with micropore™ tape (3 Micropore™, St Paul, Minnesota, USA) (after prior warning). The image intensifier is then rotated into the true lateral position (no other movement of either the x-ray equipment or the patient is allowed). The angiography table is raised or lowered until the tip of the long sheath and the bifurcation is isocentric and the full diameter of the coin is visible in the anterior-most aspect of the image. Angiography is performed in the lateral position and calibration performed.

Lesion crossing and filter deployment

(see Figure 7.19)

- An in-depth discussion of the evidence-base for cerebral protection and an exploration of the pros and cons of each type of protection device available is beyond the scope of this book. It will be assumed that a filter-type protection device is to be used.
- The projection that allows optimal vizualisation of the route through the lesion is selected.
- The lesion is crossed using a 'no touch' technique as far as possible, on road-mapping.
- The 0.014 guidewire integral to the protection device or separate (in the case of 'bare wire' systems such as the EmboShield Pro, Abbott Vascular Devices Ltd. (Farnham, Surrey, UK) and the SpideRx, ev3 Neurovascular, Irvine, California, USA) is used to cross the lesion. The tip of the wire is curved into the most appropriate shape for lesion crossing.
- Once the lesion is crossed on road-mapping, the filter is deployed (wire-mounted system) or loaded into the 190 cm guidewire (all components of the carotid stenting procedure are now rapid-exchange compatible) and deployed in the distal ICA ('bare wire' systems).

TIPS:

The CCAs are surprisingly mobile, the right slightly more so than the left. The tip of the long sheath may be seen to move up and down quite markedly in some patients, with cardiac pulsations, perhaps by as much as 1.5 cm.

When the lesion is difficult to cross, (e.g. very tight and tortuous), lesion-crossing may be timed with either systole or diastole – whichever gives the best approach to the lesion.

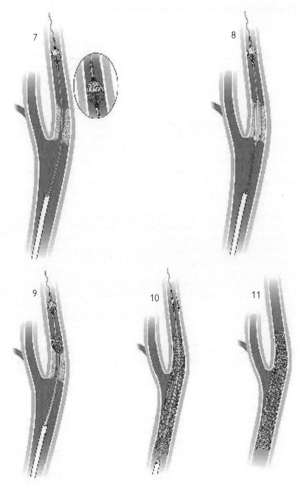

Figure 7.19 Schematic representation (7-11) of placement of the filter wire, to stenting. © Cordis.

Pre-dilation, stenting and postdilatation

(see Figure 7.18)

- Lesions tighter than around 90% have an insufficient residual luminal channel to allow unhindered passage of the stent-delivery system. Some of the larger-diameter stents have undeployed crossing profiles of around 5.9F (just under 2 mm) and these will simply not pass through a tight lesion without risk of uncontrolled embolisation ('snow-ploughing'). Predilatation with a 3 mm balloon is routinely performed for tight stenoses.

- For heavily calcified lesions, particularly those with circumferential or globular calcification, 2.5 or 3 mm cutting balloons may be appropriate prior to stent placement. It could, however, be argued that these lesions should be avoided, particularly by novices and the patient referred for the tried and tested gold standard, carotid endarterectomy, instead.

- Balloon inflation should be controlled by means of an inflation handle. Six atmospheres for around 6 secs is usually sufficient.

- 1.2 mg of atropine or 300 μg glycopyrollate (synthetic derivative of deadly nightshade with fewer tendencies to cause confusion in the elderly and cardioaccelerator effects than atropine) are administered via the long sheath prior to balloon dilatation of the carotid bulb.

- The filter-device, balloons and stent are all rapid-exchange compatible. A 190 cm 0.014 guidewire is therefore sufficiently long. All carotid equipment runs 'over the wire' for 10–15 cm or so and then the shaft of the balloon, stent etc runs parallel to the guidewire. To advance rapid-exchange-compatible equipment over this guidewire, once beyond the 'over the wire' section, the index finger and thumb of the left hand grip the guidewire at its exit point from the haemostatic valve of the long sheath, the right hand advances the balloon shaft or delivery system of the stent.

- The stent is advanced to the end of the long sheath (see Tips opposite). The stent is advanced across the lesion under road-mapping and deployed usually when the tightest point of the lesions is equidistant from the leading and trailing ends of the stent. Some operators switch road-map off at the point of stent deployment, for optimal stent visualization.

- Post-dilatation is considered to be one of the most hazardous aspects of the procedure. When the stent expands into friable plaque there is always the concern that debris is squeezed through the interstices of the stent, perhaps particularly so if the stent is forced onto the plaque by post-dilation.

- Five millimetre post-dilation is usually adequate for most patients. The incentive is not to treat 'claudication of the brain' but rather control friable plaque that is vulnerable to embolisation. A slight waist is therefore perfectly acceptable after stenting in this arterial territory.

TIPS AND CAUTIONARY TALES:

- The platinum-tip of the 0.014 guidewire is advanced as far as the radiopaque end of the long sheath. Road-mapping is then performed, allowing the patient little time to move.
- Refrain from rapidly releasing the pressure within the balloons by employing the 'quick release' mechanism of the inflation handle. This has the potential to take the carotid by surprise (which is never advisable) and risks plaque prolapse into the vessel lumen. The pressure within the balloons is steadily decreased by 'winding down' the pressure handle instead.
- Administration of atropine or glycopyrrollate via the long sheath causes unilateral mydriasis which can sometimes cause consternation amongst the nurses and junior doctors looking after the patient on their return to the ward. They should be reassured, or preferably, told in advance of this eventuality.
- Balloon-expandable stents are prone to deformation due to neck movements are to be avoided. Dedicated carotid stents are associated with a lower adverse event rate than stents 'adapted' from coronary or peripheral platforms (5).
- Before stent deployment it is important to ensure that the trailing end of the stent is not inside the long sheath (the radiopaque marker on the end of the long sheath will indicate its tip) and that the trailing end of the filter is well clear of both the lesion and the nose-cone of the stent delivery system. Impaction of the stent delivery system on the fully deployed filter is never a good look.
- Asystole is most likely to occur during post-dilatation. Asking the patient to cough will aid in restoration of heart rate, if the glycopyrrollate/atropine has not been sufficient to prevent bradyarrythmias.
- Many experienced operators tailor their stent and protection system to the patient with respect to patient anatomy, lesions characteristics, whether the patient is symptomatic or not and whether the patient has severe aortic valve disease or is awaiting coronary artery bypass grafting. Consideration of these choices is beyond the scope of this chapter and the reader is directed to the appropriate source (6).

Completion and closure

- Angiography is performed in at least two views (orthogonal) to evaluate the following:
  - That there is no plaque prolapse through the interstices of the stent (this will require magnified views of the stent on angiography).
  - That there is good filling of the distal ICA.
  - That the filter is not occluded.
  - That there is no obvious loss of intracranial vessels as a result of embolization. Those practitioners who advocate routine imaging of the intracerebral circulation post-CAS argue that these views be taken prior to manipulation of the lesion also, for purposes of comparison.

TIPS:

- Plaque prolapse: This will require low pressure (4 atmospheres) balloon dilatation for around three minutes (if the contralateral ICA is patent and the patient likely to tolerate this manoeuvre). Sometimes, despite this, another stent will need to be placed, inside the first, to 'double the scaffold'.
- No filling of the distal ICA: flow limiting spasm, dissection and an occluded filter will all cause flow arrest. Under these circumstances the distal ICA will not fill with contrast.
- Spasm is usually evident early in the procedure and gentle cephalad movement of the filter, slow administration of boluses of diluted glyceryl trinitrate 100–200 μg into the long sheath and/or prompt completion of the procedure and retrieval of the filter is likely to resolve the problem. Spasm is usually well tolerated.
- An occluded filter might require aspiration through a large-bore catheter prior to filter-retrieval.
- Dissection of the distal ICA may require additional stent placement.
- Careful evaluation of the trailing 'dot' markers or Nitinol hoop at the base of the filter may give some clues as to the cause of flow arrest. If the markers or hoop are drawn together, compared with the immediate post filter-deployment images, then dissection or flow-limiting spasm are potential causes of the problem. If there is no change in the appearance of the base of the filter, a full filter is the more likely problem.
- A closure device is routinely used to close the femoral puncture. A StarClose (extraluminal Nitinol clip) (Abbott Vascular) has the advantage of no intraluminal component and the 6F iteration will actually close the 8F hole caused by 6F long sheaths. The patient can usually sit up within around 1 hour of completion of the procedure.

After-care

- A neurological examination is carried out immediately post-procedure and neurological observations continued for at least six hours post-procedure on the ward. Pulse and blood pressure evaluations are also vitally important for a 24 hour period.
- The commonest cause of a prolonged admission (longer than 24 hours) following CAS is blood pressure derangement. The reader is directed to material highlighting the importance of periprocedural haemodynamics (7).
- In the vast majority of patients a systolic blood pressure of around 100–110 mmHg (relatively common) is well tolerated and expectant treatment is the order of the day. Nurses should be careful that such patients do not jump out of bed precipitously and faint behind a locked toilet door. The baroreceptors (responsible for lowering the blood pressure after stent deployment and postdilatation) take around 24 hours to reset themselves to baseline levels. Timely resetting of the baroreceptors is promoted by earlier mobilization (which is, in turn promoted by mechanical closure of the puncture site).

- In certain subsets, (pre coronary artery bypass or aortic valve surgery, relative hypotension may not be well tolerated and these patients may be better cared for in a High Dependency Unit (HDU) overnight. Most low cardiovascular risk patients can be cared for on an 'ordinary' ward such as cardiology, stroke medicine or vascular surgery.
- Sustained hypertension (systolic blood pressure 20% above baseline lasting at least one hour is a real cause for concern, particularly when associated with headache (which may be frontal, periorbital, migrainous, etc.) and may herald the much feared hyperperfusion syndrome and haemorrhagic stroke, which has a high fatality rate. Strenuous efforts should be made to control the blood pressure of these patients, with transfer to HDU for invasive arterial blood pressure monitoring.

TIPS:

It is not uncommon to reduce the patients' antihypertensives on discharge, with instructions to attend their General Practitioner's practice for re-evaluation of blood pressure after discharge.

The patient should be instructed to reattend if sustained headache occurs after CAS, in order to avoid hyperperfusion syndrome / haemorrhagic stroke.

References

(1) National Institute for Clinical Excellence (2006). Carotid artery stent placement for carotid stenosis. IPG 191. September 2006. London: NICE 2006.

(2) Patient selection: Anatomical Williams, R.E.T., Macdonald, S., Chapter 7, in *Carotid Artery Stenting; A Practical Guide*. Editors Stansby G., Macdonald S., Springer.

(3) Pre-procedure imaging: Van Den Berg, J., Chapter 5, in *Carotid Artery Stenting; A Practical Guide*. Editors Stansby G., Macdonald S., Springer.

(4) From: *Carotid Interventions*. Schneider P.A., Bohannon W.T., Silva M.B. (eds) (2004) Marcel Dekker, p.16).

(5) McKevitt F.M., Macdonald S., Venables G.S., Cleveland T.J., Gaines P.A. (2004) Complications following carotid angioplasty and carotid stenting in patients with symptomatic carotid artery disease. *Cerebrovasc Dis.* **17:** 28–34.

(6) Plaque stability and carotid stenting: Bosiers, M., Peeters, P., Chapter 8, in *Carotid Artery Stenting; A Practical Guide*. Editors Stansby G., Macdonald S., Springer.

(7) Relevance of periprocedural haemodynamics: Macdonald, S., Chapter 14, in *Carotid Artery Stenting; A Practical Guide*. Editors Stansby G., Macdonald S., Springer.

Methods of arterial closure

Methods of arterial closure

- Manual compression.
- Mechanical devices – e.g. Femstop.
- Surgery.
- Closure device.

Manual compression

Standard technique involves firm compression for a minimum of 10 minutes over the puncture site sometimes longer with anticoagulation, larger devices, calcification, etc.

Puncture site complications

These include:
- Haemorrhage/haematoma.
- Emboli.
- AVM.
- Pseudoaneurysm.
- Occlusion.

Advantages

- It has stood the test of time >50 years.
- It is the Gold Standard.
- No additional equipment.
- Cheap.

Disadvantages

- Time consuming.
- Bed–rest required.
- Complications are potentially serious.
- Uncomfortable for patients and operator.

Adjuncts to manual compression

These include:
- Mechanical clamp devices (femstop) and hemostatic pads. Mechanical clamp devices apply direct pressure onto the puncture site.
- Topical haemostatic pads contain procoagulants, which promote clot formation; however, these pads still require a degree of manual compression.

Closure devices

These are used increasingly following interventions. Some, however, use these routinely as they
- can reduce time to haemostasis;
- can reduce time to ambulation.

However, they have not reduced the incidence of puncture site complications.

Potentially useful

- anticoagulated patients;
- larger sheath sizes;
- poorly compliant patients.

Devices

- No perfect device or clear indication of which device to use.
- No dramatic difference efficacy/complications.
- Suture devices may have advantages with larger arteriotomies (stent grafts).
- Extravascular devices may be preferable with pvd.
- Familiarity and experience with any given device is likely to reduce adverse outcomes.

Three main types

(see Table 8.1)

- Collagen based.
- Suture based.
- External clip/staple.

Table 8.1 Availble Vasular Closure Devices (VCD) and their mechanisms of action

Device type	Manufacturer	Substrate/ mechanism	Relation of VCD to vascular wall
Sealant devices			
AngioSeal™	Daig, Minnetonka, MN, USA	Bovine collagen	Intraluminal
VasoSeal™	Datascope Corp., Montvale, NJ, USA	Bovine collagen	Extraluminal
Duett™	Vascular Solutions, Inc., Minneapolis, MN, USA	Collagen plus thrombin	Extraluminal
QuickSeal™	SUB-Q Inc., San Clemente, CA, USA	Gelatin	Extraluminal
NeoMend	MeoMend, Inc., Sunnyvale, CA, USA	Bioadhesive	Intraluminal
On-Site	Datascope Corp., Montvale, NJ, USA	Bovine collagen	Extraluminal
Suture-mediated devices			
Perclose®	Perclose®, Abbott Laboratory, Redwood City, CA, USA	Suture	Intraluminal
X-SITE™	X-SITE Medical, Blue Bell, PA, USA	Suture	Intraluminal
SuperStitch®	Suture®, Inc., Fountain Valley, CA, USA	Suture	Intraluminal
Staple-mediated devices			
EVS Vascular Closure System	Angiolink Corporation, Taunton, MA, USA	Titanium staple	Extraluminal
Starclose	Abbott Laboratory, Redwood City, CA, USA	Nitinol	Extraluminal
Others			
TheraSeal®	Therus Corporation, Seattle, WA, USA	Ultrasound	Extraluminal
Syvek Patch®	Marine Polymer Tech., Danvers, MA, USA	Cellulosic polymer and poly-n-acetyl glucosamine	Extraluminal
Cb-Sur		Polyprolate Acetate	Extraluminal
Boomerang	Cardiva Medical USA	Nitinol	Intraluminal

An example of each type is given below

Angio-Seal®

Come in 6/8F systems. Can be used to close holes of slightly larger French size (8F devices have been used in up to 12F but against manufacturer's advice).

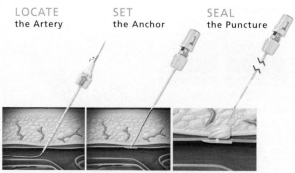

LOCATE
the Artery

SET
the Anchor

SEAL
the Puncture

Figure 8.1 Deployment of Angio-Seal® (images provided courtesy of St. Jude Medical)

- The Angio-Seal® sheath (A) is placed within the vessel via the existing guide wire.
- It is advanced until blood flows out through the exit hole in the dilator as shown.
- It is then withdrawn until the blood flow ceases and is advanced until the blood flow restarts.
- (B) Locator and guidewire are removed. The Angio-Seal® is inserted fully into the sheath with two arrows on the sheath and device assembly meeting.
- The anchor will then be released beyond the sheath tip. The barrel of the device is retracted with a double 'click' and the whole assembly
- is then withdrawn.
- The anchor will be fixed against the inside of the vessel by gentle traction.
- A tamper becomes visible on the suture as the sheath is removed.
- (C) Once fully visible, the tamper is advanced forward to tie a knot over the collagen plug, which becomes compressed against the puncture site.
- The suture is then cut above the tamper and the tamper is removed.
- Finally, the suture is cut close to the skin.

It used to be said that there should be no repuncture within 90 days. However, it is easy to puncture slighter higher or lower if necessary before then.

Perclose®

6F system. A single device has been used up to 14F by using the pre-close technique, i.e. deploying the suture at the time of gaining access, then dilating up the tract to the required size and then at the end of the procedure tying the sutures so as to close in the manner below. Using two pre-deployed devices has been successful in closing 24–25F holes following EVAR.

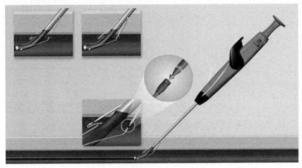

Figure 8.2 Deployment of Perclose® (images provided courtesy of Abbott Vascular).

- The sheath is removed and exchanged with the Perclose® device over a guide wire.
- When the device is within the vessel to an adequate depth, arterial blood returns from the marker lumen (arrow).
- Raising the lever deploys the footplate, which is then retracted to the vessel wall.
- The plunger is depressed, sending two needles from the sheath through the artery wall to the footplate.
- The needles engage the suture, and the plunger is withdrawn, which draws the suture out through the proximal part of the device.
- The lever is lowered so the device can be partially withdrawn and the suture/knot combination can be pulled free.
- The device is removed and the slip part of the knot (green in color) is pulled to advance the knot to the arteriotomy, aided with a knot pusher.
- The knot is then pulled tight white suture to secure the arteriotomy.
- The knot pusher also acts as the suture cutter by advancing the tab forward as clot to the knot as possible.

TIPS:

Pre-close technique for large holes, i.e. >10F i.e EVAR
- Access artery using standard seldinger technique.
- Dilate to 6F.
- Introduce perclose over the wire and rotate clockwise 10 degrees and deploy.
- Place clip on the sutures (white and green) and attach to drape the locking suture (white) to the left and slip suture (the green) right of the patient.
- Repeat with second device but this time rotate 10 degrees anticlockwise keeping the two sets of sutures apart to avoid confusion.
- Dilate to appropriate sheath size.

At procedure's end wash all the sutures carefully with saline right into the wound if possible to reduce friction and then tie the correct pair of sutures in the standard way while an assistant maintains firm pressure above puncture site to maintain haemostasis during closure.

Starclose®
An external clip, currently the 6F system, has been used in slightly larger holes against manufacturers' recommendations.

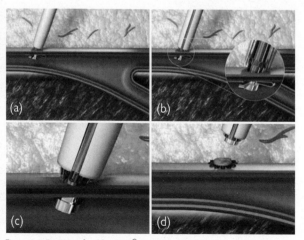

Figure 8.3 Deployment of Starclose® (images provided courtesy of Abbott Vascular).

- The procedure sheath is replaced with the star close sheath
- The StarClose® device is inserted into the sheath until it clicks in place.
- The vessel locator button is depressed.
- The device is pulled out gradually until resistance is felt (the internal vessel locater is at the internal lumen wall.
- (B) The advancement of the thumb advancer completes the splitting of the sheath.
- The device is raised to an angle of slightly less than 90 degrees.
- (C) The clip is deployed.
- (D) The device is retracted.

Outcomes
- 89.4–100% technical success.
- haemostasis 94–100%
- major complications 1.2–2%:
  - haemorrahge
  - pseudoaneurysm
  - AVM
  - occlusion/emboli (collagen devices)
  - infection

For a fuller account please see Further Reading.

Further reading

Hon, L.-Q. Ganeshan, A., Steven, Thomas, M., Warakaulle, D., Jagalpathy, J. and Uberoi, R. (2008) *Curr. Probl. Diagn. Radiol.*

Stentgrafting

Principles

Stentgrafts are usually covered with PTFE or Dacron.

Indications

- Acute vascular ruptures.
- Aneurysms.
- Symptomatic complicated aortic dissections.
- Fistulas.

They have been used in occlusive disease but there are no good data to support their use.

The self expanding type is usually used for major large vessels, i.e. aorta, iliac's. The balloon or self expanding type can be used for smaller vessels.

Renal, subclavian, and splanchnic vessels may be treated with either but are treated most often with balloon expandable stents, including ruptures. Balloon expandable stents are less frequently used.

The sizing of vessels is crucial using either CTA, MRA, or Angiography. Axial images are best for true diameters.

10–15% oversize and even 20% may be indicated by some manufacturers for self expanding stents. Size to vessel for the balloon mounted type.

Thoracic aorta

Plan case with MRA or CTA (Figure 9.1).
- Need to asses accurately diameter of landing zones i.e.:
  - Length of landing zone.
  - Total length of graft required.
  - Tortuosity of landing zones.
  - Tortuosity and diameter of iliac arteries for access.

One needs iliac arteries ideally > than the external size of the delivery, i.e. 8 mm or more, but 6.5–7 mm luminal diameter may be ok for smaller devices.

TIPS:

Uncalcified vessels will stretch up a bit. But don't push too hard. Treat stenosis well before procedure date.
Moderate tortuosity will straighten with a stiff wire, however the vessel will ruck up.
If small vessels or very tortuous consider iliac conduit or axillary approach.

Ideally one needs 2 cm of proximal and distal neck, i.e. a relatively normal aorta distal to the carotid arteries and proximal to the celiac. The subclavian may be covered, but will need a bypass to reduce risk of stroke and paraplegia.

There is an increased risk of paraplegia with a larger area of thoracic aorta cover and covering of the left subclavian artery.

Femoral access is usual with surgical cutdown. Using pre-deployment of suture closure devices can allow a percutaneous approach (see Chapter 8).

- Opacify arch aorta with 4/5F pigtail catheter in the ascending aorta either from a brachial approach or contralateral femoral in steep LAO to open arch.
- Mark position of proximal vessels, i.e. carotid on the screen or use fluoro-fade if available and distal landing zone.
- Deployment procedure varies with specific devices.
- Drop blood pressure to <90 systolic to reduce windsock of the stent during deployment.
- Deploy stent by withdrawing outer sheath to reveal half of the first stent.
- Re-opacify the arch to confirm accurate positioning.
- Re-position if necessary forward or backward.
- If satisfactory, in one smooth movement remove the whole sheath.
- If there is a locking wire this should now be removed.
- Do a final check of the angiogram to assess for endoleak in at least two planes.
- Only balloon dilate if there a leak and moulding the proximal or distal attachment will be of benefit.
- Avoid ballooning in dissections.

TIPS:

Sometimes a hybrid approach is required with re-implantation of the carotid or brachiocephalic trunk prior to stenting to give sufficient landing zone. The stent can be deployed at the same time or delayed to another session. If deploying at the same sitting in theatre one can deploy from the open proximal arch, but some devices will need to be specially modified for this.

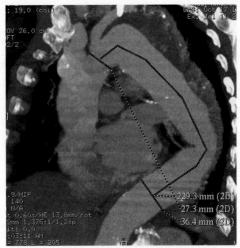

(a)

Figure 9.1a Sizing of the thoracic aorta is often best performed with CT using the axial slices for the diameter measurements (remember to allow for tortuosity and measure the true diameter i.e tangential to direction of movement) and reconstructions for length. Remember inner and outer curve measurements particularly for proximal sealing zone.

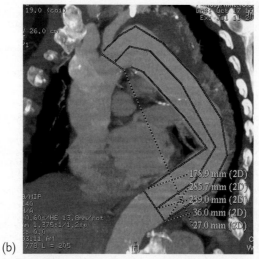

Figure 9.1b *(continued)*

Abdominal aneurysms

Usually dealt with by trouser grafts or uniliac devices; uncommonly tube grafts for the abdominal aorta only.

Plan the case using MRA or CTA (Figure 9.2) but it is more complex than thoracic cases.

- Need to asses accurately the diameter of landing zones, i.e. infra-renal neck and both common iliacs or external iliacs.
- Length of landing zones.
- Total length of graft required.
- Tortuosity of landing zones (most devices not recommended for angulations of greater than 60 degrees).
- Tortuosity and diameter of iliac arteries for access. Marked tortuosity (90 degrees) can makes access for device delivery impossible, particularly if calcified. Even if a device can be placed there is a major risk of kinking following removal of the stiff wires.

Need 15 mm neck below renal arteries or longer sealing zone if possible ideally and in the common iliac arteries.

Tube grafts of the aorta only are rare.

TIPS:

If the common iliac arteries are >23 mm one will need to extend down into the external iliac arteries. This will also require occlusion of the internal iliac arteries on the ipsilateral side. If bilateral there is a major risk of mesenteric ischemia and Leriche syndrome, consider:

- Branched graft (Figure 9.3).
- Aorto-uniliac graft with fem-fem x over graft, with stentgraft from external iliac into internal iliac artery with occlusion of common iliac above.

Procedure

- Bilateral groin cut downs, percutaneous approach less commonly used.
- Bilateral 7F sheaths placed.
- 4F straight flush catheters through separate puncture in to the CF artery to opacify the internal iliac arteries.
- 4–5 Pigtail catheter through contralateral.
- 7F sheath and opacify renal arteries and iliac bifurcation.
- Mark renals on the screen and the iliac bifurcation. Markers under the patient are useful or fluoro-fade may be useful. This can be left.
- Place stiff wire, i.e. 260 cm Lunderquist or amplatz superstiff up to the proximal thoracic aorta (avoid going into cranial vessels and heart).
- Orientate device for trousers for the correct position of the short and long limbs.
- Advance main device. Re-opacify the renals with cranio caudal angulation if forward neck angulation and centre on the renal arteries. Ensure contralateral limb is above the iliac bifurcation.
- Release device until contralateral limb exposed.

- Withdraw pigtail catheter and cannulate the contralateral limb with curved catheter, i.e. Cobra, MPA or BMC, terumo wires are helpful.

TIPS:

Keeping the ipsilateral limb attached allows some movement of the contralateral limb to help with cannulation and docking. Or if having difficulty cannulating try oblique views or use brachial approach.

- Exchange for stiff wire as above. Dock contralateral limb.
- Opacify ipsilateral internal iliac. Release ipsilateral limb so that end is just above the internal iliac artery.
- Confirm at least one and half stent overlap (ideally) of dockng of limb and place distal end just above internal iliac artery by hand flush injections into the 4F catheters .
- Use moulding balloon to open up ruffles of the graft material at sealing zones and junction of limbs.
- Extensions will be required if incorrectly sized or using Cook's tri-fab device.
- Completion angiogram in two planes to look for endoleak.

TIPS:

Aspiration through the groin sheaths will help opacify the iliacs quicker. If renals inadvertently covered it may be possible to pull the whole graft down by inflating a balloon above the bifurcation and pulling!
Or use a through and through wire over the bifurcation in the graft out of both groins and again pulling. Be careful with devices with hooks!

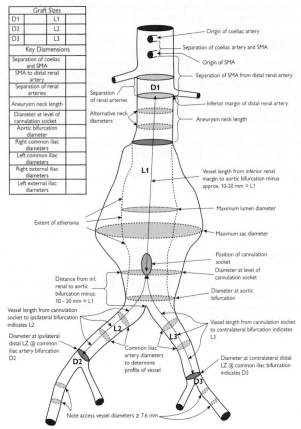

Graft Sizes		
D1		L1
D2		L2
D3		L3

Key Dimensions	
Separation of coeliac and SMA	
SMA to distal renal artery	
Separation of renal arteries	
Aneurysm neck length	
Diameter at level of cannulation socket	
Aortic bifurcation diameter	
Right common iliac diameters	
Left common iliac diameters	
Right external iliac diameters	
Left external iliac diameters	

Figure 9.2 Example of sizing sheet.
Neck length (Proximal landing zone >15mm)
Neck diameter (Up to 30–32mm with some devices)
Narrowest diameter of the aorta (often forgotten but important as limbs may not expand if too narrow i.e. <18mm)
Distance to C iliac bifurcation
Distance to I iliac bifurcation
Diameter of C iliac arteries (Up to 22mm with some devices)
Diameter of E iliac arteries (For access)
Some manufacturers also require the distance of the SMA and Celiac arteries above the renal arteries for their device (Aorfix). © Lombard.

Supra-renal and thoraco-abdominal stentgrafts

These are carried out only in specialist centre and all need special manufacturing tailored to individual patients.

Localized iliac aneurysm

(see Figure 9.3)

One needs ideally a 2 cm sealing zone above and below the aneurysm. If across the internal iliac one will need to occlude this as well to prevent endoleak.

For large common iliac arteries one can use the reversed limb of stent-graft, i.e. up to 23 mm.

Occlusion of the internal iliac for limb extension down into the external iliac artery:

Options
- Use large multiple coils, i.e. Nester or spiral.
- Use Amplatzer cheaper than multiple coils.
- Glue with or without coils.

Dealing with External iliac aneurysms (Figure 9.4):
- Will need to occlude outflow vessels using the above.
- If proximal neck >2 cm may try amplatzer plug.
- If neck <15 mm use stentgraft across the internal iliac artery from the common iliac to external iliac artery.

Renal, subclavian and splanchnic vessels may be treated with either but most often with balloon expandable stents, including ruptures.

Follow up patient with pre-discharge, 3 month and annual imaging thereafter, i.e. duplex, MR but most commonly CT.

TIPS/Caution:
- Don't routinely balloon post stent grafting in dissections due to risk of extension of the dissection.
- Immediate post procedure angiogram should be in two planes to help identify leaks. Newer C arms have rotational or CT abilities which is extremely valuable.
- If a type 1 leak (proximal attachment) is identified, it needs immediate treatment. Try ballooning for 1 minute up to 3 times. Proceed to placing a large Palmaz stent (Figure 9.5) if leak persists over neck to fully expand the graft.
- If still leak persists will require a proximal extension cuff.
- If type II leak identified this can be followed up as long as the sac does not enlarge. Majority will seal on follow up.
- If the renal arteries are covered this will require urgent renal revascularization. Successful attempts at pulling the device down have been performed, i.e. using the moulding balloon inflated at the bifurcation or a wire across the bifurcation and out both groins and pulled down. These carry considerable risk.
- If both internal iliacs are accidentally covered these may not necessarily result in long term (particularly if diseased) symptoms but ideally should be avoided.

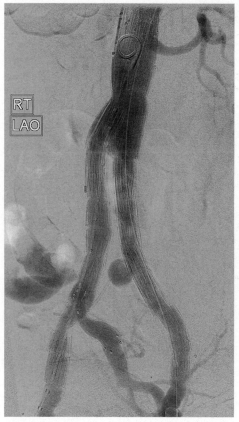

Figure 9.3 Branched stentgraft with an internal iliac branch to allow extension of graft into both external iliac arteries and preservation of one internal iliac artery.

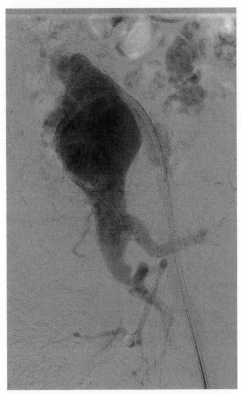

Figure 9.4a Occlusion of an internal iliac artery aneurysm using an Amplatzer device. Note the aneurysm has displaced the bifurcation up.

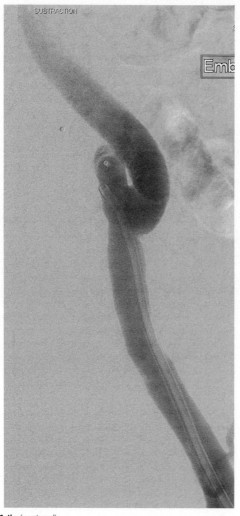

Figure 9.4b *(continued)*

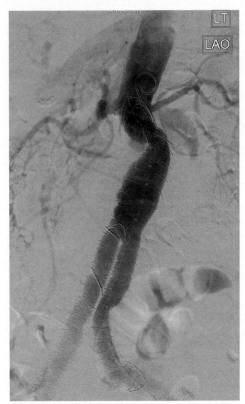

Figure 9.5a Type 1 endoleak following and Aorfix stentgraft in a very tortuous neck >80 degrees.

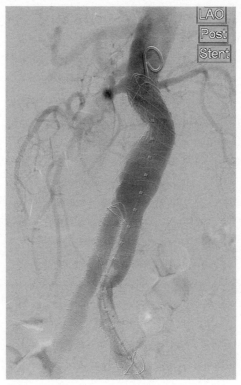

Figure 9.5b Successfully treated using a large Palmaz stent.

Interventional radiology in transplantation

Introduction

Orthotopic liver transplantation (OLT) has become the treatment of choice for patients with end-stage non-malignant liver disease and in patients with early stage hepatocellular carcinoma (HCC). Although survival rates of over 80% at one year have been reported, it remains a technically challenging procedure and its success is highly dependent upon the correct selection of patients before transplantation and the accurate diagnosis and treatment of complications after the procedure. The commonest liver transplantation procedure is the whole organ OLT. The shortage of available donor organs has led to innovative techniques of reduced-size 'split' liver and living related liver transplantation.

Interventional radiology before transplantation

The main aim of pre-OLT imaging is to evaluate the vascular anatomy in living- related donors. Advances in cross-sectional imaging particularly multi-detector computed tomography (MDCT) provide excellent information on vascular anatomy as well as liver volumetric assessment and has virtually replaced the need for invasive angiography. Hepatic angiography in donors is performed in the small number of patients in whom MDCT has failed to depict the vascular anatomy.

Hepatic angiography

- Standard common femoral arterial puncture under local anaesthesia.
- Use a curved 0.35 guidewire (Storq™ or standard 'J') and advance the wire into the aorta.
- Replace the puncture needle with a 5F sheath.
- Introduce a 5F Sidewinder™ catheter over the wire and advance the catheter to the arch of aorta with the wire leading the catheter.
- Withdraw the wire into the descending aorta and twist the catheter so that it resumes its pre-determined shape.
- Pull the catheter down the aorta with its 'nose' facing anteriorly.
- Advance the tip of the catheter into the coeliac axis; confirm position with 2–5 mls of contrast.
- Inject contrast with a pump injector (30–40 mls of contrast at 6–8 mls per second) to obtain images of the arterial tree.
- It is important to visualize the left gastric artery as 10–20% of patients will have a replaced or accessory left hepatic artery arising from the left gastric artery.
- Push the catheter up so that it disengages from coeliac axis. Twist the catheter slightly so that the nose points away from coeliac axis and pull it down.
- Once the catheter has gone past the coeliac axis turn its nose anteriorly to catheterize the superior mesenteric artery; confirm position with 2–5 mls of contrast.
- Inject contrast with a pump injector (same volume and rate as above) to evaluate accessory or replaced hepatic arterial vasculature and indirectly evaluate the superior mesenteric vein and portal vein (prolonged imaging).

TIPS:

- **Sidewinder™ does not form in the aortic arch:** This may happen in patients with tortuous iliac arteries and an ectatic aorta. Remove the Sidewinder™ and use either a Sos Omni™ or Cobra™ catheter.
- **Cannot catheterize the coeliac axis:** This may happen when there is coeliac axis stenosis or atheromatous plaque in the aorta. Do not use force; try a different catheter (Sos Omni™, Cobra™).
- **Cannot see the left gastric artery:** This usually indicates that the tip of the catheter is distal to the origin of left gastric artery (LGA). Withdraw the catheter by pushing it up so that the tip lies in the proximal coeliac axis.
- **There is an accessory supply from the LGA but this is not adequately opacified:** Selectively catheterize the LGA artery with a Sos Omni™ catheter and a hydrophilic guidewire (Terumo™ or Roadrunner™) and hand inject contrast.
- Sometimes it may be necessary to use a co-axial micro-catheters (Progreat™ or Renegade™) to catheterize small accessory hepatic arteries and perform contrast injections with pump at low volume and pressure (20 mls at 3 mls per second)

Interventional radiology post liver transplantation

(see also 📖 Chapter 3 and 📖 Chapter 4)

The surgical techniques and immunosuppressive therapy for liver transplantation have improved considerably. Nevertheless, there are still significant complications, particularly those of vascular origin, which can lead to graft failure and require re-transplantation unless prompt treatment is instituted. These complications include arterial and venous thrombosis and stenosis; arterial pseudoaneurysm; biliary leakage, stricture and obstruction; liver ischemia, infarction and abscess formation; fluid collections and haematoma formation.

The clinical presentation of post transplantation complications are frequently non-specific and vary widely; imaging studies are critical for early diagnosis. Ultrasound (US) is normally an accurate, non-invasive method of demonstrating hepatic vessels (hepatic artery, portal vein, hepatic veins, and inferior vena cava) and evaluating non-vascular complications (in the hepatic parenchyma and bile duct abnormalities) and extra-hepatic tissues. MDCT is a valuable complement to US in the post-operative period. Knowledge and early recognition of these complications is essential for graft salvage, and MDCT can provide valuable information, particularly for patients with indeterminate US results or in whom the US examination is difficult.

Hepatic artery thrombosis

Hepatic artery thrombosis (HAT) is the most common and significant vascular complication, and accounts for approximately 60% of vascular complications post-liver transplantation. Clinical presentation varies from delayed, intermittent episodes of septicemia or abnormal liver function to fulminant hepatic failure. Doppler US is able to detect up to 92% of cases of HAT. Definitive diagnosis of HAT requires evaluation with MDCT angiography or conventional angiography. Complete occlusion of hepatic artery often requires surgical intervention or re-transplantation.

Hepatic angiography

- Prior to arteriography it is vital that the interventional radiologist to be fully aware of the surgical vascular anastomoses that were performed in the patient.
- The initial technique is identical to that described above. Use a Sos Omni™ or a Cobra™ catheter and place the tip of catheter in the coeliac axis. Gently inject 10–20 mls of contrast by hand.
- In cases where an infra-renal arterial conduit graft is used, perform a lateral abdominal aortogram with a pigtail catheter. This allows adequate delineation of the graft origin and can be followed by selective graft catheterization with a Cobra™ or Sos Omni™ catheter.

TIPS:

Avoid using a guidewire to catheterize the coeliac axis as it may be difficult to differentiate guidewire associated spasm/dissection from stenosis/occlusion.

Hepatic artery stenosis

In the majority of patients, hepatic artery stenosis (HAS) occurs at the surgical anastomoses and is linked to technical factors, clamp injury, kinked vessels, fibrosis, oedema and thrombus formation. Non-anastomotic stenosis may be secondary to allograft rejection or clamp injury. Early recognition and intervention may help prevent significant ischemic organ damage and progression to HAT. In cases of HAS a Doppler US may demonstrate a focally accelerated velocity (greater than 2.0 m/second) and turbulent flow at and beyond the anastomoses. A tardus-parvus waveform is seen downstream from the stenosis with a sensitivity and specificity of about 75%.

Hepatic artery angioplasty

(see Figure 10.1)
- Perform standard coeliac axis angiography with a 6F sheath and Sos Omni™ catheter to define the anatomy and locate the stenosis.
- Using a standard Storq™ guidewire parked carefully in the coeliac axis; replace the catheter with a 6F guide catheter.
- Use a low profile (4 mm × 2 cm) balloon catheter mounted on 0.18″ guidewire to catherterize the hepatic artery via the guide catheter.
- Cross the stricture with the guidewire followed by the balloon and dilate the stenosis gently to the recommended pressure.
- Deflate the balloon and inject contrast through the guide catheter and repeat the inflation if necessary.

TIPS:

- Always use a guide catheter and a low profile (4 mm or 5 mm diameter) short balloon (2 cm) to negotiate the tortuous artery.
- Give heparin and isosorbide mononitrate prior to crossing the stricture and after the angioplasty if necessary.
- Never use force and do not use high pressure as there is a risk of rupture.
- In case of difficulty in crossing the stricture or advancing the guidewire further into hepatic artery use a hydrophilic guidewire (0.18 Terumo™).

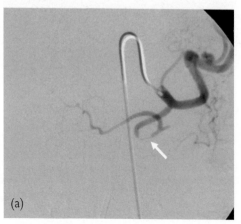

(a)

Figure 10.1 a) Selective angiography of coeliac axis demonstrating a conventional arterial anastomoses with a short segment stricture (arrow).

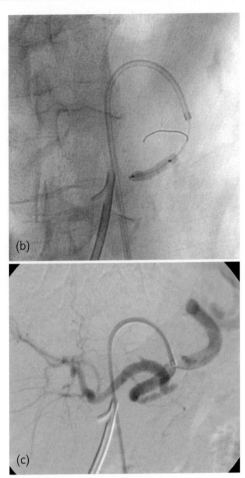

Figure 10.1 b) Balloon dilatation of the hepatic artery stenosis with a 5mm balloon.
c) Post balloon dilatation images demonstrating a patent hepatic artery and good
arterial inflow into the graft.

Hepatic artery pseudoaneurysm

(see Figure 10.2)

Hepatic artery pseudoaneurysm (HPA) formation and arteriovenous fistula represent less common arterial complications post-liver transplantation. These may be due to surgical anastomotic breakdown from technical factors, infection or may be related to post-transplantation iatrogenic injuries such as percutaneous biliary drainage or biopsy. HPA may be treated by percutaneous (thrombin injection) or by endovascular techniques such as embolization or by placement of an arterial stent graft. The surgeons should be consulted prior to the intervention as it may have an impact on further surgical management and vascular reconstruction.

Embolization of HAP

- Perform diagnostic angiography to establish the diagnosis and suitability for safe coil embolization without compromising the arterial inflow to the graft.
- Use a co-axial micro-catheter (Progreat™) to catheterize the aneurysm.
- Place the catheter tip beyond the neck of the aneurysm. Gently deploy 0.18″ coils (2–3 mm) into the aneurysm carefully ensuring the coils do not reflux into the main hepatic artery.
- Perform gentle contrast injections to ensure that the aneurysm is sufficiently packed with coils and the main hepatic artery stays patent.

TIPS:

Do not use very small coils as there is a danger of displacement and reflux into the main hepatic artery.

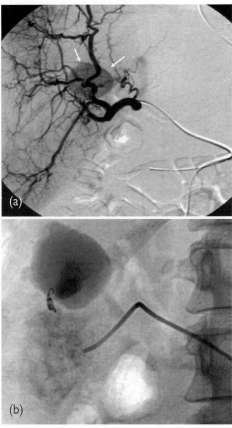

Figure 10.2 a) Selective angiography of hepatic artery demonstrating a pseudo-aneurysm (arrows) arising from a segmental branch close to the hilum. b) Embolization of the feeding artery with 2mm coils.

Portal vein complications

Portal vein stenosis is an uncommon complication with a reported incidence of 3% in adults and 7% in children. Stenosis usually occurs at the site of the surgical anastomoses and may be related to surgical technique, a redundant vein or the use of a bypass graft. Patients may be asymptomatic, present with portal hypertension or with abnormal liver function tests on routine blood biochemistry. Diagnosis can be made with Doppler US or MDCT.

Portal vein venoplasty

(see Figure 10.3)

- Portal vein access via a trans-hepatic, trans-jugular or trans-splenic approach. Trans-hepatic approach is preferred.
- Position the patient supine on the angiography table with right arm placed on a horizontal armrest.
- Using fluoroscopy or US to mark a suitable area on the skin in the mid-axillary line at a level of the liver hilum.
- Infiltrate the skin, subcutaneous tissue and the liver capsule with adequate local anaesthetic.
- Make a small incision in the skin and introduce a 23G Chiba™ needle into the liver parenchyma.
- Remove the stylus and connect the needle to a syringe containing contrast via a connector tube with a 3-way tap.
- Inject contrast and gradually withdraw the needle. Identify a suitable portal venous radical and introduce a short 0.18″ guidewire.
- Gently manipulate the guidewire into the main portal vein.
- Replace the Chiba™ needle with an introduction sheath system (Neff™ or modified Gould™ system).
- Inject a small amount of contrast confirm the venous position and replace the introduction sheath with a 7F sheath (or larger depending on the balloon size required) via a Storq™ 0.35 guidewire.
- Introduce a short 65 cm multi-purpose catheter over the wire and cross the stricture. Place the catheter in the superior mesenteric vein (SMV) and perform venography to outline the anatomy and the length of the stricture.
- Flush the catheter and connect it to pressure manifold and measure the pressure gradient across the stricture. If the stricture is haemo-dynamically significant then proceed to angioplasty.
- Replace the catheter with a 10 mm or 12 mm balloon and perform venoplasty.
- Confirm successful dilatation with venography and repeat dilatation with a wider 14 mm balloon if necessary.
- Check the pressures again to ensure there is no pressure gradient across the stricture.
- In patients with recurrent stenosis it may be necessary to stent the anastomoses. In which case a 12 mm or 14 mm wide and 4 cm or 6 cm long self-expanding metallic stent can be used.
- Perform venography to demonstrate the anatomy. Select a suitable reference image and note the position of the meso-splenic vein confluence.
- Place the lower end of the stent proximal (nearer liver) to the meso-splenic vein confluence in order not to occlude the splenic vein.
- Balloon the stent gently to allow expansion at the site of the stenosis (moulding). Perform venography to ensure patency of the SMV, splenic vein and portal vein.
- Withdraw the catheter into the sheath first and gently withdraw both while embolizing the puncture tract with gelfoam or PVA particles.

TIPS:

- While puncturing the portal vein with a Chiba™ needle do not cross the liver hilum in order to avoid damage to the hepatic artery
- Use a 4F dilator to manipulate the 0.18 wire into the main portal in case of difficulty in tracking the wire.
- In case of a tight stricture do not force the wire as it may dissect the portal vein.

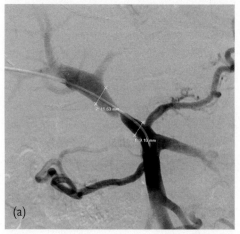

Figure 10.3 a) Direct trans-hepatic portal venography demonstrating a short segment stenosis of the extra-hepatic portal vein at the level of the anastomoses.

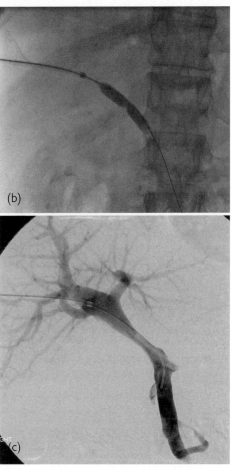

Figure 10.3 b) Venoplasty with a 10mm balloon. Note the 'waisting' of the balloon at the site of the stricture. c) Venography post balloon dilatation confirms a successful procedure with no residual stricture.

Hepatic vein stenosis

Hepatic venous stenosis has a reported incidence of 4% in post-transplant patients and is more common in split liver grafts. Patients present with ascites and a 'Budd-Chiari-like' syndrome with biochemical hepatic dysfunction. Diagnosis can be made on Doppler US and biopsy often shows passive venous congestion. Endovascular management with balloon dilatation is the first line of management. Recurrent stenosis can be treated with endovascular stent placement. A stenosis may also occur in the IVC, with similar endovascular options available (Figure 10.4).

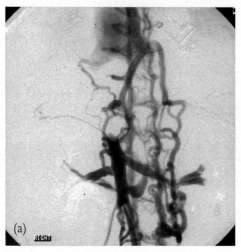

Figure 10.4 a) Venography of a left lobe split graft with IVC stenosis and hepatic venous outflow obstruction with an occluded hepatic segment of the cava and prominent venous collateral drainage.

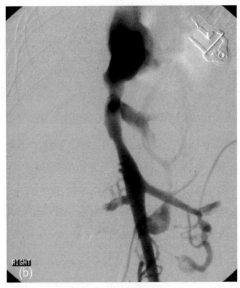

Figure 10.4 b) Venography following balloon dilatation of the IVC demonstrating successful recanalization.

Hepatic vein venoplasty

- Right internal jugular or common femoral vein approach can be used. Trans-jugular approach is often preferred as it is technically easier to access the hepatic veins particularly in patients with a 'piggy-back' anastomoses.
- Place a 5F sheath in the right internal jugular vein. Introduce a standard 'J' or Storq™ guidewire into the SVC.
- Introduce 4F short (65 cm) multipurpose catheter over the guidewire. Manipulate the wire and the catheter into inferior vena cava (IVC).
- Catheterize the right hepatic vein initially and advance the guidewire into the hepatic vein as distally as possible. Advance the catheter over the guidewire.
- Remove the guidewire and perform venography to demonstrate the anatomy.
- Evaluate the stricture and measure the pressure gradient across the stricture and measure the pressures in IVC and right atrium.
- If there is a haemo-dynamic significant stricture then proceed to venoplasty.
- Exchange the multi-purpose catheter with a short 4 cm balloon (6 mm to 10 mm diameter) and dilate the narrowed segment of the hepatic vein.
- Perform check venography to confirm satisfactory dilatation and repeat the procedure if necessary.
- In case of a recurrent stricture a self-expanding stent may be used. Use an extra-stiff or ultra-stiff Amplatz™ guidewire to provide greater stability. Use a 4 or 6 cm long stent (6–8 mm diameter) and place it cross the stricture. Balloon dilate to mould the stent.
- If there is a stricture in the proximal aspect of the hepatic vein close to the IVC, take due care to place the stent so that the proximal end of the stent lies flush with hepatic venous orifice and does not protrude into IVC.

TIPS:

- In case of difficulty in catheterizing the hepatic vein use a Cobra™ catheter and a long sheath to provide greater stability.
- In case of a tight stricture in the proximal hepatic vein a trans-jugular biopsy introduction device may be used taking due care and avoiding injury to anastomoses.

Biliary intervention

(see Figure 10.5)

Biliary tract complications post-liver transplantation have a reported incidence of 15% and are often due to surgical technique or hepatic arterial insufficiency secondary to hepatic artery stenosis or thrombosis. Normally in liver transplantation, a duct to duct anastomoses or a Roux-en-Y biliary enterostomy are performed. When biliary intervention is required, an endoscopic approach is difficult in patients with Roux–en-Y biliary enterostomy and requires a percutaneous approach under imaging guidance.

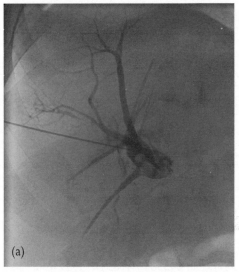

(a)

Figure 10.5 a) Percutaneous cholangiogram demonstrating dilated intra-hepatic ducts with a tight anastomotic stricture and debris proximal to the stricture.

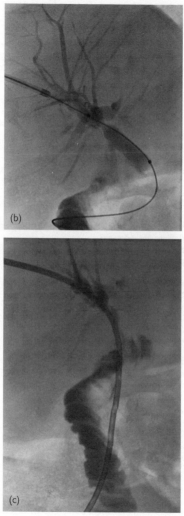

Figure 10.5 b) A guide wire crosses the stricture and balloon allowing dilatation of the stricture with 10mm balloon. c) Post-procedure cholangiogram and placement of internal–external biliary catheter drain.

Percutaneous trans-hepatic cholangiography (PTC)

- Place the patient supine on the angiographic table with the right arm extended and placed on an arm support.
- Mark a suitable area on the skin using fluoroscopic guidance or US guidance and puncture a suitable bile duct with a 23G 15 cm Chiba™ needle.
- Perform a cholangiogram to demonstrate the anatomy and confirm the presence of stricture.
- Introduce a 0.18 guidewire through the Chiba™ needle and manipulate the guidewire into main common hepatic duct.
- Replace the needle with an introduction sheath (Neff™ or modified Gould™ sheath).
- Replace the 0.18 wire with a 0.35 guidewire (Storq™ or standard 'J' guidewire).
- Replace the introduction sheath with a 6 or 7F sheath.
- Use a short (65 cm) 4F multi-purpose catheter and manipulate the guidewire across the stricture into Roux-en-Y loop.
- Replace the multi-purpose catheter with an 8 mm or 10 mm balloon catheter and dilate the stricture.
- Remove the balloon and perform a cholangiogram through the sheath to confirm patency of the anastomoses and repeat the dilatation if necessary.
- Remove the balloon and sheath and place an 8F internal external biliary drain cross the stricture.
- Secure the drain to the skin with a suture or appropriate dressing.
- Practices vary; it is generally advisable to leave the biliary catheter on free drainage for 24 to 48 hrs depending on the severity of jaundice.
- Perform a tubogram in 1 week and re-dilate the anastomoses if required.
- It is generally advisable to leave the internal-external biliary drain in place for 4 to 6 weeks and repeat the tubogram. If there is a recurrent stricture then the patient would require biliary reconstruction surgery.

TIPS:

- A 0.18 guidewire will not advance: replace the Chiba™ needle with a 4F dilator to support the guidewire.
- Unable to cross the stricture at first attempt: place an external biliary drain to relieve the jaundice and attempt to cross the stricture at a later date.
- Unable to introduce the internal-external biliary drain: this can be problem particularly with left bile duct punctures; dilate the track or use a peel-away sheath over an ultra-stiff Amplatz™ guidewire.

Renal transplantation

Introduction

Renal transplant complications can be managed by minimally invasive techniques but are more challenging than interventional procedures in the native kidney. The most common procedure performed in the transplant kidney patient is a biopsy of the graft; histology important in the management of episodes of rejection. Other procedures performed include drainage of collections, nephrostomy with ureteric dilatation and stenting and balloon dilatation of a transplant renal artery stenosis.

Renal biopsy

A biopsy procedure is normally straightforward and differs little from biopsy of the native kidney except the target organ is more superficial and readily visualized.

- Place the patient supine on a couch, and assess the kidney with ultrasound, choosing a site for biopsy away from major vascular structures.
- An adequate core biopsy should contain cortex and medulla.
- Real time guidance of the biopsy needle should be performed.
- Use a 16 or 14 gauge biopsy needle, complications include arteriovenous fistulae, arterio-calyceal fistulae and pseudoaneurysm formation.

> **TIPS:**
>
> Use a transvenous route or a 'plugged' biopsy if an uncorrectable coagulopathy is present.

Fluid collection drainage

Fluid collections are common and include lymphoceles, urinomas, haematomas, and abscesses. These may occur in up to 18% of renal transplant patients. Small collections do not require treatment and may be watched. Techniques for percutaneous drainage are similar to drainage procedures elsewhere.

- Place the patient supine on a couch, and assess the kidney with ultrasound
- Drain larger collections with a pigtail catheter (8–16F) under ultrasound guidance, insert a second drain if needed for a large collection.
- Use either the trocar or Seldinger technique, under real time control with ultrasound.
- Use a 'stiff' guidewire, e.g. Amplatz Stiff or Ultrastiff, as the surgical procedure makes the subcutaneous tissues more difficult to pass a catheter.
- Lymphoceles may require prolonged drainage.

> **TIPS:**
>
> - A locking pigtail will prevent inadvertent removal.
> - Flush the drainage catheters regularly to prevent blockage

Renal obstruction and nephrostomy

Occurs in 2–10% of transplant patients with early obstruction, often a consequence of operative oedema and a late stricture, a consequence of ischaemia at the distal aspect of the transplant ureter. Leakage at the distal ureter may be managed with nephrostomy and stent, and a stricture with balloon dilatation prior to stent placement. Most nephrostomy procedures may be performed electively unless sepsis is evident or serum potassium levels are dangerously elevated.

- Place the patient supine on a fluoroscopy couch, and assess the kidney with ultrasound.
- Selection of an appropriate calyx will minimize radiation exposure to the operator's hands and allow ease of passage of guidewire down ureter to enter the bladder if needed.
- Use a 22 gauge Chiba needle to puncture a calyx, aspirate some urine for microbiology, and inject some diluted contrast to confirm position in the collecting system.
- A 0.0018 guidewire is inserted and followed by a transitional dilator and stiffener, e.g. Neff Set.
- Remove the stiffener and inner dilator, and pass a 0.035 guidewire.
- Dilate the tract to 8F and position a locking pigtail catheter.

TIPS:

- The original 0.0018 guidewire may be left in place to prevent inadvertent position loss whilst manipulating catheters.
- Surgical changes may necessitate the application of a stiff guidewire to position the nephrostomy catheter.

Ureteric balloon dilatation and stenting

Normally a nephrostomy is established a few days prior to a dilatation or stenting procedure.

- The original nephrostomy allows passage of a guidewire (usually a stiff angulated hydrophilic guidewire) across the ureteric stricture to the bladder.
- Placement of a 9F peel-away sheath provides secure access across the scar tissue.
- A dedicated ureteric stent for renal transplants is used.
- The stent is advanced over the guidewire with the pusher, and position secured with the protruding Ethilon suture, which is removed once stent positioning is satisfactory.
- If the stent cannot be advanced across the ureteric stricture, a balloon (5–6 mm) can be used to dilate the stricture.
- A nephrostomy should be left in place especially if there is haematoma from the procedure within the collecting system (Figure 10.6).
- The ureteric stent may be removed via a cystoscopy 6–8 weeks after placement.

TIPS:

- Allow the pigtail to reform freely in the bladder prior to removal of the guidewire; failure of reformat suggests that the distal end of the stent remains in the ureter.
- Reposition the upper end of the stent using the Ethilon suture, then cut and remove this; buttress the stent against the peel away sheath to prevent movement as suture is removed.

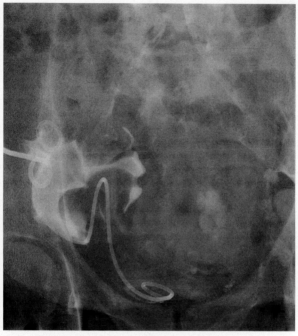

Figure 10.6 Percutaenous nephrostomy followed by ureteric stent.

Renal artery stenosis

Renal artery stenosis is reported to occur in up to 30% of patients. This is often the result of surgical clamp injury, but may also arise due to cyclosporine toxicity, donor atherosclerosis and vessel kinking. The clinical sequelae are hypertension and renal failure. Endovascular treatment is preferable to surgical repair and may be either subject to balloon dilatation or stent placement.

- Place a 5–6F sheath and use an appropriate catheter (usually a Sos-Omni) to access the transplant renal artery.
- A tapered tip guidewire (TADII or a Roadrunner) is used to cross the lesion.
- Use a short length (2 cm) balloon (5–7 mm) to dilate the stenosis.
- Use a stent only if the vessel collapses following balloon dilatation or a dissection is seen (Figure 10.7).

TIPS:

A cadaveric graft (external iliac anastomosis) is accessed from the ipsilateral approach and a live donor graft (internal iliac anastomosis) from a contralateral approach.

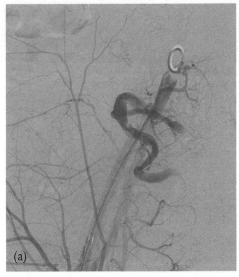

(a)

Figure 10.7 a) Stenosis in the renal artery resulting in poor renal function and hypertension.

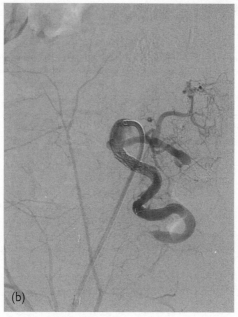

Figure 10.7 b) Post dilatation and stenting.

Pancreas transplantation

Pancreatic transplantation is not a life-saving procedure but allows for the control to glycaemia and control of progression of complications. The majority of pancreas transplants are performed in conjunction with a simultaneous renal transplant. Most transplants are performed with endocrine drainage into the systemic venous system and exocrine drainage into the urinary bladder or into the bowel to avoid complications associated with bladder drainage. Vascular thrombosis of the pancreatic transplant occurs in 12% (5% arterial) of patients (Figures 10.8–10.9), and allograft pancreatitis may develop. Complications may also arise in the simultaneous renal transplant.

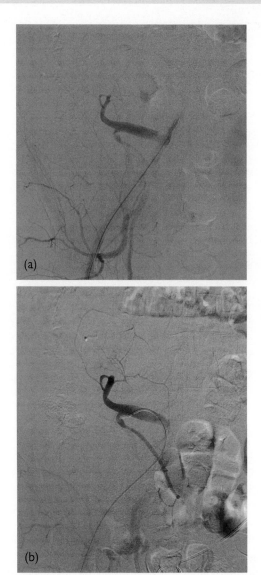

Figure 10.8 a) Acute occlusion of pancreatic transplant artery b) Following thrombolysis.

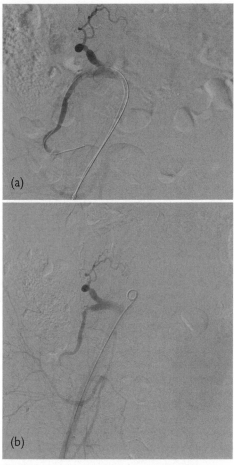

Figure 10.9 a) Pancreatic transplant artery stenosis b) Post stenting.

Islet cell transplantation

This minimally invasive technique has grown in popularity over the last 5 years with improved Islet cell recovery from cadavers, culturing techniques and percutaneous instillation into the portal vein. The patients still require full immunosuppresion.

Indications

Patients with brittle diabetes and failure of conventional insulin therapy.

Contra-indications

- Portal hypertension or thrombosis.
- Bleeding diathesis.

Preparation

- Consent/Clotting/FBC/U/E/LFT/Cross match.
- IV access.
- Monitoring O_2/ECG/ Pulse/BP.
- Usually fasted for 4 hrs.
- Sliding scale for diabetic control glucose infusion.
- Commence immunosuppressants.
- Antibiotics.

Equipment

- Neff/Acustics set (Mandril wire/other).
- Dilater.
- 4F long sheath (23 cm).
- C Arm/US.

Technique

- Procedure almost identical to PTC (see 📖 Chapter 13) (Figure 10.10).
- Procedure performed in Radiology suite under conscious sedation.
- Under US control right distal anterior Portal branch ideal target is punctured.
- A 0.18 mandril wire or V18 control wire is advanced into the portal vein and parked in the distal splenic vein.
- A 4 F sheath is placed distal to the main portal vein bifurcation.
- Check portal pressure <12 mmHg.
- Portogram to assess anatomy (Figure 10.10).
- Islet cells mixed with dextran 40 in 0.9% sodium chloride and 35 units heparin per kg body weight.
- Propriety kits which contain a Chiba needle, 0.018 wire, and sheath/dilator are useful i.e. Neff, Accustix etc
- Slow gravity infusion.
- Thromboelastogram (TEG) monitoring of venous samples during procedure.

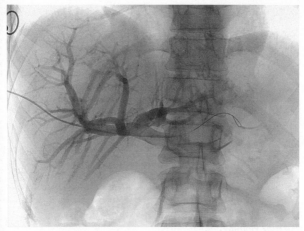

Figure 10.10 Portogram following successful portal cannulation using a Neff set under US and Fluoroscopic control.

- Intermittently check portal pressure, maintain <12 mmHg.
- Completion portogram and pressures.
- Embolize tract Spongiostan/coils (Figure 10.11).
- Monitor on dedicated ward, i.e HDU/transplant ward.
- Pulse/BP/Resp every 15 mins for 4 hours, then half hourly for 4 hours.
- Continue sliding scale.

Complications
- Bleeding/haematoma.
- Portal vein thrombosis (major cause for failure on early transplants).
- Sepsis.
- GB puncture.
- Next day US/MR to assess portal patency and look for bleeding.
- Continue anti-rejection drugs.
- Discharge when medications stabilized, i.e. 3–5 days.
- Follow up with US/MR 3/12.

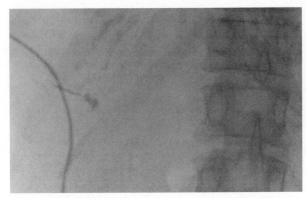

Figure 10.11 Embolization of the tract at the end of the procedure with gelfoam mixed with some contrast.

Further reading

Almusa O., Federle M.P. (2006) Abdominal imaging and intervention in liver transplantation. *Liver Transplantation* **12**: 184–193.

Amesur N.B., Zajko A.B. (2006) Interventional radiology in liver transplantation. *Liver Transplantation* **12**: 330–351.

Hobart M.G., Streem S.B., Gill I.S. (2000) Renal transplant complications. Minimally invasive management. *Urol. Clin. North Am.* **27**: 787–798.

Quiroga S., Sebastia C., Margarit C, Castells L., Boye R., Alvarez-Castells A. (2001) Complications of orthotopic liver transplantation: spectrum of findings with helical CT. *RadioGraphics* **221**: 1085–1102.

Interventional uro-radiology

Percutaneous nephrostomy

This is one of the most commonly performed interventional procedures and is frequently performed in the out-of-hours clinical setting. Knowledge of applied renal anatomy and the principles of percutaneous access is crucial in order to minimize complications.

Indications

- **Temporary urinary diversion** to relieve ureteric obstruction by ureteric calculus or pelvic malignancy (e.g. prostate carcinoma).
- **Urinary access for endourological intervention:** PCNL, ureteric stent insertion, pyeloureteroscopy, direct infusion of chemotherapy).
- **Other indications**: Urinary diversion for the management of urinary fistulas or ureteric leak, Pyosepsis, Hydronephrosis of the transplant kidney or in the pregnant patient.

Contraindications

- No absolute CIs.
- Relative:
  - Bleeding diathesis (can be corrected with FFP or Vit K).
  - Uncooperative patient.

Patient preparation

- Consent.
- Bloods FBC/U&Es/clotting.
- IV access and rehydrate if necessary.
- NBM at least 4 hrs prior to procedure.
- Stop any medication that may predispose to haemorrhage (e.g. aspirin, warfarin, NSAID).

Procedure

> **TIP**
>
> ❶ Review prior imaging to gain idea of approach to kidney.
> ☛ Always safer to perform procedure during working hours as there is lower risk of complications. Only proceed out-of-hours if urgent clinical need, e.g. pyosepsis/single kidney.

- Medication:
  - Sedation: midazolam (1 mg boluses);
  - Analgesia: fentanyl (25 mg boluses);
  - Antibiotics: single dose, prior to start of procedure, according to local guidelines (e.g. gentamicin/cephalosporin).
- Patient positioned prone or prone oblique on fluoroscopy table.
- Sterile preparation including ultrasound probe cover.
- Re-image kidney with U/S to plan access approach.
- Infiltrate skin and soft tissue with 1% lidocaine. Deeper infiltration also advisable – a 20G spinal needle can be used.
- 5 mm skin nick is made.

Single puncture technique

This is reserved for significantly dilated pelvi-calyceal systems where urgent drainage is required and future ureteric access unlikely to be needed.

- Advance introducer needle through the soft tissues and cortex of kidney under direct U/S visualization.
- A 21G access needle (e.g. Accustix) is the safest choice to minimize risk of bleeding but larger calibre sheathed needles (e.g. 16G Kellett needle) can be used for very dilated collecting systems.
- With needle tip positioned adjacent to calyx advance needle 10–15 mm with short stabbing motion – a 'pop' can usually be felt indicating access to collecting system.
- Once access is confirmed (dilute contrast can be injected) advance guidewire under careful fluoroscopic control.
- If a 21G needle was used to advance the dilator/sheath component over the 0.018 wire and exchange for a standard 0.035 wire. The guide-wire should ideally be placed down the ureter (a 5F Cobra catheter and hydrophilic wire can be used) but the procedure is still possible with the wire curled up in the upper collecting system.
- Serial dilation of the tract to 1F greater than the nephrostomy catheter.

TIPS:

- Always use fluoroscopic guidance to prevent kinking of wire.

- Insert nephrostomy catheter (most commonly 8F pigtail catheter) into collecting system. Withdraw wire until 'pigtail' forms and position in renal pelvis. Lock the catheter and fix to skin with silk suture. Or fixation device.

Double puncture technique

Overall a safer technique that aims to ultimately access the safest calyx, usually a mid/lower pole posterior calyx. Can be performed in the minimally dilated kidney and is the procedure of choice for endo-urological access.

- Direct ultrasound puncture of collecting system with 21/22G needle – inject dilute contrast to delineate calyceal anatomy.
- Inject air to identify posterior calyces – these with become more lucent than the contrast filled anterior calyces.
- Position the most suitable posterior calyx directly in the centre of the image intensifier field of view.
- Make another skin nick and advance second introducer needle towards the calyx. Forceps can be used to advance the needle and to keep the operator's hand out of the x-ray beam.
- Once the needle enters the kidney (will move in synchronicity with the kidney with respiration) angle the gantry at least 20 degrees in oblique direction to obtain depth information.
- Line up needle with the calyx and advance into the collecting system. Return the gantry to the AP position and confirm successful access with injection of contrast. Repeat steps above if not successful.

- As with the single puncture technique insert guidewire into ureter (may need to upgrade to standard wire via use of sheath/dilator) and perform serial fascial dilatation.
- Insert nephrostomy catheter (as above).

Pitfalls

- If urine is aspirated but guidewire doesn't follow – the needle tip is against the calyceal wall and needs careful re-positioning
- If the guidewire kinks during access don't persevere and 'push harder'- rather exchange for a stiffer wire (e.g. Amplatz super stiff).

TIPS:

Take care not to lose access!

For nephrostomy insertion in the pregnant patient avoid the use of radiation and perform under ultrasound guidance only. For this reason the procedure is more technically challenging and should only be performed by an experienced operator and ideally during working hours. Alternatively, consider urological options, e.g. retrograde stent insertion under GA.

Complications

- Haemorrhage; minor bleeding is almost guaranteed in the form of haematuria but should settle within 24 hrs. Major bleeding requiring transfusion, surgery or embolization occurs in 1–4% of cases.
- Sepsis – more common if nephrostomy performed to relieve blocked infected system (therefore minimize injection of contrast to prevent bacteraemia!).
- Urine extravasation.
- Pneumothorax.
- Visceral injury – colon, gall bladder.
- Inability to remove catheter due to crystallization – catheters should be removed or exchanged after 3–4 weeks.
- Mortality rate <0.3%.

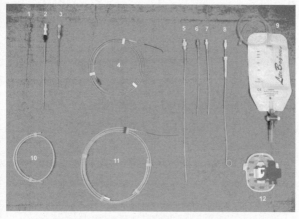

Figure 11.1 Equipment required for percutaneous nephrosotmy.

1. Chiba type needle.
2. Sheathed dilator set which comes with the Skater or Accustick introducer set.
3. Kellet needle.
4. 0.35 Hydrophylic wire, i.e. Teruma.
5. Angled catheter i.e. Biliary Manipulation catheter (BMC).
6. 6F dilator.
7. 8F dilator.
8. Pigtail drainage catheter.
9. Drainage bage (leg catheter drainage bag).
10. 0.18 wire (Cope- Mandril, etc.).
11. Amplatz superstiff.
12. Fixation device, i.e. Drain fix.

Further reading

American College of Radiology – Practice guideline for the performance of percutaneous nephrostmy (ww.acr.org/SecondaryMainMenuCategories/quality_safety/guidelines/iv/percutaneous_ nephrostomy.aspx).

Major complications after percutaneous nephrostomy-lessons from a department audit (2004) *Clin. Radiol.* **59**(2): 171–9.

Patel, U. and Hussain, F. (2004) Percutaneous Nephrostomy of Nondilated Renal Collecting Systems with Fluoroscopic Guidance: Technique and Results. *Radiology* **233**: 226–33.

Percutaneous renal access for PCNL

PCNL is the treatment modality of choice for the removal of complex renal stones. It is highly effective with success rates of up to 98% for renal stones and 90% for ureteric stones. PCNL comprises of four stages:

- Cystoscopy and retrograde ureteral acess.
- Percutaneous renal access.
- Tract dilatation.
- Stone removal. The procedure of percutaneous renal access is described here as this is performed typically by an interventional radiologist.

Indications

- Renal calculi >2 cm.
- Staghorn calculus.
- Lower pole stone >1 cm.
- Abnormal renal anatomy (e.g. horseshoe kidney/calyceal diverticulum)
- CI/ Failure ESWL.
- Calcium oxalate monohydrate/cystine stones.
- Calculi associated with infundibular, PUJ or ureteral obstruction.
- Failure of conventional treatment.

Contraindications

- No absolute CIs.
- Relative CIs:
  - Co-morbidity preventing general anaesthesia in the prone position (e.g. obesity).
  - Active/untreated infection urinary tract.
  - Coagulopathy.
  - Severe kyphoscoliosis precluding adequate approach.
  - Pregnancy.

Patient preparation

- Recent imaging demonstrating location of stones and pelvicalyceal anatomy (MDCT with 3D volume rendered reconstruction is ideal, good quality IVU is adequate).
- Bloods: FBC/ U&Es/clotting.
- ECG.
- CXR.
- Cannula.
- Consent.
- Nil per mouth 4–6 hours before procedure.
- Stop any medication that may predispose to haemorrhage (e.g. aspirin, warfarin, NSAID).

Equipment

- **Entry needle:** 22G access systems 4F/5F sheathed diamond tip needle (e.g. Kellett)/18G Nephrostomy needle.
- **Guidewire:** 0.035 standard J tip wire/ 0.035 J tip hydrophilic wire/ 0.035 super-stiff wire.

- **Catheters:** 5–6F shaped tipped catheter(e.g. Cobra/ Kumpe/BMC).
  Dialtors: telescopic metallic/ sequential teflon (Amplatz)/balloon.
- **Working sheath** 24–34F.

Calyx selection

- The goal of PCNL is complete stone clearance. If this is not possible aim to:
  - clear the renal pelvis/PUJ to allow drainage of the collecting systems;
  - clear the lower pole calyces (not easily treatable with ESWL). Select a calyx with these aims in mind.
- A Posterior Calyx is preferable to an anterior calyx due to a lower risk of arcuate/lobar artery injury and easier intrarenal navigation.
- A posterolateral approach into a lower pole calyx is the safest as it passes through a relatively avascular plane and avoids the pleural cavity, however visualization of adjacent lower pole calyces may be impossible.
- Carefully chosen upper pole entry will allow complete clearance of the lower pole calyces, renal pelvis, PUJ and upper ureter.

Fluoroscopically guided calyx puncture

- Opacify collecting system with contrast medium (injected via retrograde ureteric catheter).
- Consider use of CO_2/air which preferentially fills posterior calyces in the prone patient, providing negative contrast.
- An angled needle approach to the calyx allows more favorable calyceal entry and navigation. Position the C-arm accordingly (Figure 11.2).
- The calyx chosen for access should be placed in the iso-center of the radiograph monitor to minimize guidance errors due to beam divergence.
- Position the needle so that calyx, needle tip, and needle hub are in line ('bull's eye' configuration on screening monitors).
- Advance needle in small increments maintaining a bull's eye configuration.
- When the needle pierces the renal capsule ($\approx$7-10 cm depth) the needle tip will be seen to move with the kidney on respiration.
- Aim to puncture the selected calyx at its center through the relatively avascular plane between the anterior and posterior divisions of the renal artery (Brödel's line).
- Check the depth of the calyx by angling the C-arm away by 20 degrees and advance the needle into the calyx.
- If final conformation is required that the needle is in the calyx, under continuous screening, rotate the arc from +30° to -20 degrees. The needle tip and calyx should move in synchrony (e.g. no parallax error).
- Remove the inner stylette of the needle and, if the position is satisfactory, urine will flow.
- Insert a hydrophilic wire through the needle and manipulate this down the ureter.
- Remove the entry needle and insert a shaped catheter. Through this exchange the standard wire for a super-stiff wire which is secured in the ureter.
- At this point consider inserting a second 'safety wire' adjacent to the catheter in case of lost renal access.

- Make a 1 cm incision next to the superstiff wire and dilate along the tract. Insert the working sheath (24–34F) using a rotating motion.
- Ultrasound guided calyceal puncture is performed in a similar fashion.

Pitfalls

- Punctures above the 11th rib have a high morbidity from pneumothorax and pleural collections.
- The calyx can be tough and may deviate the needle off trajectory.
- Urine back flow through needle may not be seen if the calyx is filled with CO_2/Air.
- Always use a stiff wire for tract dilatation as it straightens the orientation of the calyx, pelvis and ureter.

Complications

- Minor complications 10–25%.
- Major complications 2–7%:
  - Septic shock 0.5–3%;
  - Severe acute haemorrhage 1% (secondary to arterial tear);
  - Delayed haemorrhage (AVF formation/ pseudo-aneurysm);
  - Chest complications: Pneumothorax/empyema/effusion;
  - Organ injury: bowel/liver/spleen.

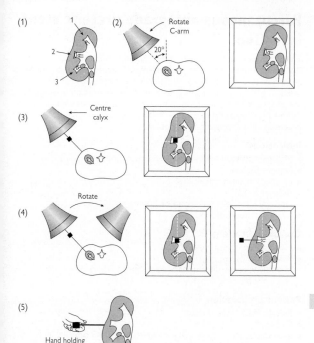

Figure 11.2 (1) The calyx is chosen according to stone location (calyx 2 for this illustration). (2) The C-arm is moved to 20° near-oblique position (with additional cranial or cephaled movement as necessary to allow an angled calyceal entry. (3) The C-arm is shifted so the target calyx is seen iso-centric and the needle hub as a 'bulls-eye' the needle slowly advanced (1cm increments) using intermittent fluoroscopy, all the while maintaining iso-centricity and the bull-eye view. (4) When the needle is seen to move with the kidney, the C-arm is moved to 20° far-obliquity. The needle image is seen to change from a bulls-eye to an angled view. The needle tip is just within/short of the calyx and requires final adjustment. (5) The side-to-side shutters are closed so that the hand on the needle hub is not in the radiation beam, and under continuous fluoroscopy the needle is advanced the final 1–2cm into the calyx. Redrawn from Patel U, Ghani K, and Anson K. *Endourology A Practical Handbook* 2006, with permission of Taylor & Francis.

Further reading

American Urological Association. Clinical Guidelines Ureteral Calculi (http://www.auanet.org/guidelines/uretcal07.cfm).

European Association Urology. Guidelines Ureteral Calculi (http://www.uroweb.org/nc/professional-resources/guidelines/online/.

Patel, U., Ghani, K. and Anson, K. (2006) *Endourology. A Practical Handbook*. Taylor & Francis.

Percutaneous antegrade ureteric stent insertion

This is a well established technique in the treatment of both benign and malignant ureteric strictures. It is minimally invasive, avoids the need for general anaesthetic, and may be possible where retrograde insertion has failed. In patients requiring long term relief of obstruction ureteral stents are preferable to nephrostomy as they are not associated with the complications of external drainage (e.g. requirement for urine bag, leakage, skin infection), thus improving quality of life.

Indications
- Malignant strictures (this is by far the most common indication).
- Benign strictures.
- Obstructing ureteric calculus.
- Adjunct to ESWL.
- Ureteral injury due to surgery or trauma.
- Ureteric fistula/leak.

Contra-indications
- No absolute contra-indications.
- Relative:
  - Active/uncontrolled urinary tract sepsis.
  - Untreated coagulopathy.

Patient preparation
- Bloods: FBC/ U&Es/clotting
- Consent
- Intravenous access (preferably minimum of an 18G cannula)
- Nil per mouth 4–6 hours before procedure.
- Stop any medication that may predispose to haemorrhage (e.g. aspirin, warfarin, NSAID).

Equipment
Guidewires: 0.035 standard J tip wire/ 0.035 J tip hydrophilic wire/ 0.035 Amplatz super-stiff wire.
- **Catheters:** 5–6F shaped tipped catheter (e.g. Cobra/Kumpe).
- **8F JJ stent:** Consists of an inner plastic cannula, a pusher catheter and the stent. The length used is determined by patient height. In general a 22 or 24 cm stent will be suitable in most patients.

Procedure
- Medication:
  - Sedation: midazolam (1 mg boluses).
  - Analgesia: fentanyl (25 mg boluses).
  - Antibiotics: single dose, prior to start of procedure, according to local guidelines (e.g. gentamicin/cephalosporin).
- Patient positioned prone.
- Access is gained to the kidney in the manner described for percutaneous nephrostomy. A posterior facing lower pole clayx is preferred but if this is felt to be unfavourable for ureteric manipulation (e.g. an acute infundibulo-pelvic angle) then a mid-pole calyx may be selected.

- If a nephrostomy is already present this can be used to gain access to the collecting system.
- A 0.035 standard wire is inserted into the renal pelvis and a catheter passed over the wire.
- Dilute contrast can be injected at this point to define the anatomy of the ureter and level of obstruction.
- The standard wire is exchanged for a curved tip hydrophilic wire.
- Wire and catheter are then manipulated past the obstructing lesion and into the bladder.
- Once the catheter tip is adequately located in the bladder the hydrophilic wire is exchanged for a stiff wire, which is coiled in the bladder.
- The ureteric stent system is assembled and inserted over the guide-wire (be careful not to inadvertently withdraw the stiff wire). The distal stent marker should lie within the bladder and the proximal end should be positioned within the renal pelvis.
- If the stent does not pass freely into the ureter, consider dilatation of the percutanous tract (using 8F/9F dilators or a 4F balloon dilator) and/or use of a peel away-sheath.
- The guidewire and inner catheter are withdrawn releasing the stent
- Maintain forward pressure on the pusher to prevent proximal migration of the stent.

TIPS:

It is very important that the guidewire is not completely removed from the renal tract, the distal end should be left within the pelvis as this maintains renal access.

- Check adequate drainage via the stent with injection of contrast.
- Check no bleeding from the percutaneous tract before removal of the guidewire.
- If there has been bleeding during the procedure and there is clot in the collecting system insert a nephrostomy tube which can be removed after 24–48 hrs.
- If a stent is for long term drainage it should be exchanged cystoscopically every 6 months..
- Metal stents can also be used. Most devices are permanent and their durability is poor. Transitional cell hyperplasia leads to blockage, with a stent life of 6–12 months.

Pitfalls
- Undersizing stent.
- Releasing the stent either too far or too proximal.

Complications
- **Common:**
  - irritative bladder symptoms;
  - supra-pubic and loin pain;
  - haematuria (microscopic/macroscopic);
  - urinary tract infection;
  - malposition;

- migration;
- inadequate relief of obstruction;
- encrustation (deposits of urine contents can form on the stent leading to blockage and possibly ureteral injury during stent removal).
- **Uncommon:**
  - stent fracture;
  - ureteral erosion.

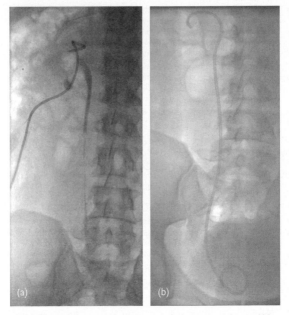

Figure 11.3 a) Nephrostogram demonstrating calculus in proximal ureter b) Image demonstrating appropriate positioning of stent

Further reading

Dyer, R. et al. (2002) Percutaneous Nephrostomy with Extensions of the Technique: Step by Step. *RadioGraphics* **22**: 503–25.

Patel, U. and Abubaker, Z. (2004) Ureteral Stent Placement without Postprocedural Nephrostomy Tube: Experience in 41 Patients. *Radiology* **230**: 435–42.

Seymour, H. and Patel, U. (2000) Ureteric Stenting-Current Status. *Semin. Intervent. Radiol.* **17**: 351–66.

Percutaneous balloon dilatation of ureteral strictures

Balloon dilatation is a straightforward treatment for benign ureteric strictures. The outcome post-treatment is variable with long-term success rates (patency at 1 year) being quoted between 48–88%. It is generally worth attempting in the first instance as the alternative usually involves surgery (endoureterotomy/ureteric reimplantation).

Indications
- Benign strictures (e.g. post ureteral instrumentation for stone removal/urteral injury during surgery/ uretero-enteric anastamotic strictures/ strictures of renal transplant ureter/post DXT/passage or calculus/ infective).
- Transplant ureteric strictures.

Contraindications
- Absolute:
  - Malignant strictures are best treated by stenting for the remainder of the patient's life.
- Relative:
  - Active/untreated urinary tract sepsis.
  - Untreated coagulopathy.

Patient preparation
- Bloods: FBC/U&Es/clotting.
- Intravenous access (preferably minimum of an 18G cannula
- Consent.
- Nil per mouth 4–6 hrs before procedure.
- Stop any medication that may predispose to haemorrhage (e.g. aspirin, warfarin, NSAID).

Equipment
- As for nephrostomy.
- **Guidewires:** 0.035 standard J tip wire/0.035 J tip hydrophilic wire/0.035 super-stiff wire.
- **Catheters:** 5–6F shaped tipped catheter (e.g. Cobra/Kumpe/BMC).
- **8F Double J stent.**
- **High pressure (8–30 atm) balloon catheter** (5–8 mm diameter/2–4 cm length).

Procedure
- Medication:
  - Sedation: midazolam (1 mg boluses).
  - Analgesia: fentanyl (25 mg boluses).
  - Antibiotics: single dose, prior to start of procedure, according to local guidelines (e.g. gentamicin/augmentin).
- Patient positioned prone and percutaneous access to the collecting system is obtained.
- Inject dilute contrast to define number, level and extent of strictures.
- Using a catheter and hydrophilic guidewire (a number of combinations may be required) cross the stricture and advance the catheter into the bladder.

- Exchange the guide wire for a 0.035 superstiff wire.
- Manipulate the balloon over the wire and across the stricture so that the tightest portion of the stricture lies at the middle of the balloon (two radio-opaque markers indicate the position of the balloon).
- Inflate the balloon slowly to the desired pressure aiming to abolish the waist (gentle counter traction or forward pressure on the balloon may be required to prevent slippage). Do not exceed manufacturer's recommended inflation pressures.
- Optimal duration and number of dilatations is debated, however 3, 1–2 minute dilatations are usually adequate.
- Resistant strictures may require the use of a cutting balloon.
- Site a ureteric stent for 3–6/52, to act as a temporary splint and to protect the ureter.

Complications

- Rupture of ureter.
- Failure – more likely in longstanding, long strictures of ischaemic aetiology (e.g post DXT/ureteric reimplantation).

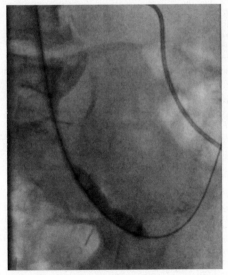

Figure 11.4 Image demonstrating balloon dilatation of uretero-enteric stricture. Note waisting.

Further reading

Dyer, R. et al. (2002) Percutaneous Nephrostomy with Extensions of the Technique: Step by Step. *RadioGraphics* **22**: 503–25.

Johnson D., Oke E. et al. (1988) Percutaneous Balloon Dilatation of Ureteral Strictures. *A.J.R.* **150**: 131–4.

Renal biopsy

(see 🕮 Chapter 19)

Indications
- Renal failure.
- Nephrotic syndrome.
- Glomerulonephritis.
- Failing transplant kidney.

Contraindications
- *Absolute*
  - Small scarred kidneys.
  - Severe polycystic kidney disease.
- *Relative*
  - Bleeding diathesis.
  - Hypertension.
  - Renal mass.
  - Pyelonephritis.

Patient preparation
- Bloods: FBC/U&Es/clotting.
- Intravenous access (preferably minimum of an 18G cannula).
- Consent.
- Nil per mouth 4–6 hrs before procedure.
- Stop any medication that may predispose to haemorrhage (e.g. aspirin, warfarin, NSAID).

Equipment

Procedure

> **TIPS:**
>
> ❶ *Review previous renal imaging (U/S, IVU or CT).*

- Performed in prone position.
- Sterile technique.
- Ultrasound guided biopsy is the most commonly used method but CT can be used (for complicated cases, e.g. biopsy of renal mass).
- Using ultrasound identify target area for biopsy: preferably upper or lower poles.
- Infiltrate with local anaesthetic from skin to renal capsule.
- Advance core biopsy needle (14–18G) into kidney and take 2–3 biopsies.
- Apply direct pressure over wound and monitor for bleeding.
- Following the procedure patient should be on strict bed rest for up to 8 hours with BP and pulse monitoring. Analgesia may be required.
- Laparoscopic and transjugular renal biopsy are additional techniques that are available but are reserved for complicated and exceptional cases.

TIPS:

❶ *Procedure can be performed on an outpatient basis or as an in-patient, however at least 8–24 hrs monitoring is required following biopsy.*

Complications
- Haemorrhage: Common following biopsy. This usually manifests as hae-maturia, and typically resolves within 24 hours. More severe blood loss can occur and may necessitate blood transfusion or even nephrectomy (<1% of cases). Mortality rate is low (<0.01%).
- Infection.
- Arteriovenous fistula.
- Pneumothorax.
- Visceral injury.

Percutaneous radiofrequency ablation of renal tumours

(see 📖 Chapter 18)

RFA achieves tumour destruction by thermally induced coagulative necrosis at temperatures of 50 to 110°C. A growing body of evidence indicates that RFA is an effective treatment for small renal tumors (3–5 cm diameter). The rate of tumour eradication ranges from 79–97% in the literature. Serious complications occur in ≈1%.

Indications

- High risk surgical candidates.
- Patients with solitary kidney unsuitable for nephron sparing surgery.
- Herditary (e.g. Von Hippel-Lindau)or non-herditary multifocal tumours.
- Patients with advanced disease to relieve symptoms related to the primary tumour.
- Patients refusing surgery.

Contraindications

- No absolute.
- Relative CIs.
  - Coagulopathy.
  - Sepsis.
  - Large tumour (no absolute limit that excludes patient from RFA ablation, however it is unlikely that complete ablation can be achieved for tumours larger than 5 cm).
  - Tumour close to major vessels or collecting systems.

Patient preparation

- Recent imaging studies.
- Bloods: FBC/U&Es/clotting (INR <1.4)/ECG/CXR.
- Cannula (preferably minimum 18G).
- Consent.
- Nil per mouth 6 hrs before procedure.
- Stop any medication that may predispose to haemorrhage (e.g. aspirin, warfarin, NSAID).

Equipment

- Commercially available RFA systems consist of an **electric generator, needle electrode** and **grounding pads** (no one system is of proven superiority).
- Needle electrodes consist of an insulated shaft and an active tip. Electrodes can be single, multiple (cluster) or have multiple retractable prongs. Size ranges from 17G–14G (no evidence at present to suggest advantage of one type of needle electrode design over another).
- Electric generators apply an ≈500 Khz AC current. Power ranges from between 150–250 W. Energy deployment can be impedance regulated or time and temperature regulated.

Procedure

> **TIPS:**
>
> ❶ *Use CT for image guidance* as this has several advantages over US:
> - Allows visualization of tumour and adjacent structures.
> - Inadvertant thermal injury to adjacent organs can be anticipated and steps taken to minimize the risk.
> - Detection of procedure related complications.

- **Conscious sedation** with fentanyl and midzolam (dose titrated to patient requirement) or **general anaesthetic** (allows control of ventilation therefore facilitating greater accuracy of probe placement.
- 24 hrs of prophylactic broad spectrum antibiotic cover (according to local prescribing policy).
- Patient positioned prone or lateral decubitus.
- Ensure grounding gel pads applied to thighs/back.
- RFA electrode is placed within the tumour in the same fashion as described for image guided biopsy.
- Biopsy can be performed prior to treatment if it is felt the results may impact on treatment and assessment of outcome.
- Once the RF probe is confirmed to be in the correct location RF energy is applied. The duration of RF treatment depends on the size of the tumour and the RFA system used.
- Aim to treat a volume slightly larger than the tumour size to ensure complete ablation.
- If a large tumour is being treated, perform initial ablation at interface of the tumour with the normal kidney (allows partial devacularization of the tumour reducing effect of perfusion mediated tissue cooling). Multiple overlapping ablations can then be performed.

> **TIPS:**
>
> ❶ *A minimum of 5 mm intervening fat should be present between bowel and the target tumour for safe ablation. If depth of fat less than 5mm consider hydrodissection to displace intestine away from tumour. Under CT guidance introduce a 22G needle between bowel and tumour and inject 5% dextrose(100–1000 mls).*

- At the end of the procedure the percutaneous tack should be thermally ablated to prevent tumour seeding.
- 24 hrs observation post procedure.
- CECT 5–7 days post procedure to assess treatment adequacy (CT prior to this is unreliable).

Pitfalls

- Flowing blood can adversely affects the size of the ablation zone (cooling effect of renal blood flow should not be underestimated).
- Tumours with a central component may be more difficult to eradicate.
- Temperatures above 105°C char tissues and decrease the effective depth of penetration of RFA.

Complications
Rate of serious complication estimated at 1%.
- Haematuria (usually self limiting and resolves within 24 hrs. Urinary obstruction may occur).
- Peri-nephric haematoma (usually self-limiting and rarely requires treatment).
- Retro-peritoneal haemorrhage.
- Penumothorax.
- Anterior abdominal wall paraesthesia or muscle weakness.
- Neuropraxia of genitofemoral n. or lumbar n.
- Ureteric stricture/PUJ stricture.
- Bowel damage.
- Release of catecholamines from adrenal glands when ablating tumours in close proximity to adrernal glands.
- Residual (unablated tumour).
- Needle track seeding.

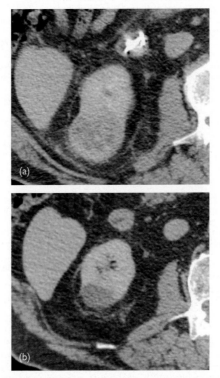

Figure 11.5 Contrast enhanced MDCT demonstrating RCC: (a) pre- RFA and (b) 2 months post RFA.

Further reading

Gervais D et al. (2005) Radiofrequency Ablation of Renal Cell Carcinoma: Part 1, Indications, Results, and Role in Patient Management over a 6-Year Period and Ablation of 100 Tumors. A.J.R. **185**: 64–71.

Gervais D et al. (2005) Radiofrequency Ablation of Renal Cell Carcinoma: Part 2, Lessons Learned with Ablation of 100 Tumors. A.J.R. **185**: 72–80.

Renal abscess

An uncommon but potentially life threatening condition that usually occurs 2 degrees to ascending urinary tract infection, often with a predisposing condition (see below). Other causes include bacteraemic seeding or direct inoculation, e.g. following instrumentation or trauma.

Predisposing conditions
- Recurrent UTI.
- Obstruction 2 degrees to calculus, tumour, or other mechanical cause.
- Iatrogenic.
- Diabetes.
- Vesico-ureteric reflux.
- Xanthogranulomatous pyelonephritis (XGP).

Radiologic diagnosis
- **Abdominal X-ray:** May show an underlying calculus or evidence of air within the collecting syste, renal silhouette, or surrounding fascial compartment.
- **Intravenous urogram**: Usually not indicated as not as sensitive as U/S or cross-sectional imaging.
- **U/S:** Look for hypoechoic renal mass usually peripheral. Underlying abnormality may be evident, e.g staghorn calculus. Important to evaualute for hydronephrosis.
- **CT:** Gold standard for diagnosis of abscess and presence of underlying condition. Scan should be performed pre and post intravenous contrast. Look for hypodense peripheral lesion. Often wedge shaped with peripheral enhancement. Main differential diagnoses include renal infarct or renal tumour.

Management
- **Medical management:** Parenteral antibiotics along with supportive measures such as IV fluids and analgesia.
- **Percutaneous drainage:** U/S or CT guided drainage. Can perform initial diagnostic aspirate, e.g. with thin gauge needle and proceed to larger drainage catheter. May need more than one catheter. Aspirate to dryness. If abscess secondary to obstructing calculus patient may need nephrostomy insertion at same time.
- **Surgical management:** Performed infrequently due to effectiveness of percutaneous techniques. Reserved for difficult cases. In certain circumstances nephrectomy may be necessary following initial percutaneous drainage, e.g. XGP.

Pitfalls
Ensure that the suspected abscess is not a tumour as RCC can present with pyrexia. If in doubt perform a diagnositic aspirate first.

Complications
- Septicaemia, multi-organ failure, and death.
- Spread into perinephric space, or even beyond into peritoneal or pleural spaces.
- Fistula formation, e.g with GI tract.
- Bleeding.

Urinary tract fistula

An uncommon condition with diverse aetiology, clinical presentation, and management. Fistula can occur at any level of the urinary tract and communicate with neighbouring structures such as the GI tract, vascular system, lymphatics, chest cavity, genitals and skin. Imaging can be complex and usually more than one investigation is required.

Causes

- **Iatrogenic:** Nephrostomy, PCNL, ESWL, abdominal surgery, vascular surgery, pelvic surgery (including hysterectomy), suprapubic cystostomy urethral surgery.
- **Infection:** XGP, urinary tract TB, parasitic infections, diverticulitis, pelvic abscess.
- **Neoplastic:** Malignancy involving urinary tract, bowel, reproductive tract; metastases, lymphoma.
- **Trauma:** Penetrating injury, pelvic fracture.
- **Other:** Radiation, Crohn's disease.

Imaging approach

- Plain radiography and ultrasound are good starting points in the imaging algorithm but rarely clinch the diagnosis. Targeted imaging modalities include:
- **Upper tract:** IVU, pyelography, ureterography.
- **Lower tract:** Cystogram, urethrogram.
- **Fistulography:** Direct visualization of fistula when feasible, e.g. cutaneous types.
- **Cross-sectional imaging:** Usually performed in conjunction with the above techniques. CT useful for both upper and lower tract imaging whereas MRI tends to be used in lower tract imaging. With CT late phase imaging is crucial.

Management

- **Treat underlying cause:** This may lead to resolution of the fistula, e.g. surgery/radiation for tumour, antibiotics for infective cause.
- **Urinary diversion:** Useful for upper tract fistulas. Either nephrostomy or stent or both,
- **Surgery:** Fistulectomy, removal non-functioning kidney, urinary diversion,
- **Embolization:** Arterial approach used in fistulas between urinary tract and vascular system. Subcutaneous embolization using tissue glue,
- **Urinary occlusion:** Only utilized in intractable/palliative cases. Can be performed surgically or percutaneously.

Further reading

Titton, R. et al. (2003) Urine Leaks and Urinomas: Diagnosis and Imaging-guided Intervention. *Radiographics.* **23**: 1133–47.

Suprapubic cystostomy

Drainage of the bladder via a suprapubic route is a common procedure in both the acute and chronic clinical setting. There are three main circumstances where suprapubic access is required:

- **Acute setting:** e.g. urgent bladder drainage where urethral drainage is contraindicated or tecnically impossible. This is commonly performed in the A&E dept and utilizes a small bore trocar guided device (e.g. 'Bannano' catheter) and is blindly inserted into a palpable bladder,
- **Surgical cystostomy:** simple technique (most commonly indicated in chronic bladder outflow obstruction) but carries risk of GA and open surgical access.
- **Image guided cystostomy:** similar indications as the surgical technique but performed under local anesthetic with/without sedation. Procedure described below.

Indications for image guided suprapubic cystostomy

- Bladder outflow obstruction (where surgery contraindicated).
- Obesity.
- Scarred lower abdomen.
- Neurogenic bladder.
- Pelvic mass.
- Radiation cystitis.
- Vesico-colonic or -vaginal fistulae.

Contraindications

- **Absolute:** Bladder tumour – especially where the intended tract may traverse tumour. This may cause a long term vesico-cutaneous fistula.
- **Relative:** Neobladder; abdominal wall cellulitis.

Patient preparation

- Bloods: FBC/U&Es/clotting.
- Intravenous access (preferably minimum of an 18G cannula).
- Consent.
- Stop any medication that may predispose to haemorrhage (e.g. aspirin, warfarin, NSAID).

Equipment

Procedure

- Medication:
  - Sedation: midazolam (1 mg boluses).
  - Strong analgesia is not usually required.
- Patient positioned supine.
- Infiltrate skin with local anesthetic.
- Distend the bladder with contrast to capacity – either by inserting a urethral catheter or by passing a 20G spinal needle into the bladder under U/S guidance.
- Make definitive puncture of bladder under U/S guidance using a 18–19G sheath needle or arterial needle.
- Under fluoroscopic guidance place a 0.035 superstiff guide wire into the bladder lumen.

- With enough wire coiled up inside the bladder the tract is dilated with serial dilators or with the use of an inflatable balloon catheter.
- Insert a peel-away sheath that is 2F larger than the intended Foley catheter.
- Cut the tip off the Foley catheter (16–20G sizes available) and pass over the wire into the bladder.
- Remove the peel-away sheath, inflate the Foley balloon and pull snugly against the anterior abdominal wall.
- The wire can now be removed. No sutures or fixation device required.
- Alternatively, once the bladder is full, use a one stick suprapubic bladder catheter system.

Pitfalls

- Ensure there are no loops of bowel between the bladder and the abdominal wall.
- Place catheter in midline through the avascular linea alba, just above the pubis.

Complications

- **Haematuria:** common, will almost always resolve.
- **Skin infection:** may require antibiotics if indicated.
- **Bowel perforation:** uncommon with the advent of image guided techniques.
- **Long term complications:** recurrent UTI and stone formation.

Further reading

Kaufman, J. and Lee, M. (2003) *Vascular and Interventional Radiology: The Requisites.* Mosby.

Lee, M. *et al.* (1993) Fluoroscopically Guided Percutaneous Suprapubic Cystostomy for Long-term Bladder Drainage: an alternative to surgical cystostomy. *Radiology* **188**: 787–9.

Renal trauma

Injury to the kidney is seen in ≈5% of patients with blunt abdominal trauma. By accurately grading the renal injury, and thereby distinguishing patients that can be managed conservatively from those that require surgical treatment, the radiologist can have a significant impact on patient outcome. The imaging modality of choice in renal trauma is MDCT.

Indications for imaging evaluation

- Penetrating injury and haematuria (microscopic or gross).
- Blunt trauma associated with haematuria (microscopic or gross) and hypotension.
- Consider the presence of injuries associated with renal trauma such as L-spine fracture/transverse process fracture/lower rib fracture.

MDCT Technique

- **Intravenous contrast medium:** 100–150 mls of a solution of 320 mg of iodine per ml with injection rate of 2–4 ml/s.
- **Section thickness:** evaluation of renal parenchyma 2.5–4 mm, evaluation of renal vasculature 0.5–1.25 mm, evaluation of rest of urinary tract 1.5–3 mm.
- **Beam pitch** of 1-1.5 mm.
- **Image acquisition:**
  - Corticomedullary phase (60–80 secs after contrast administration) to evaluate renal parenchyma.
  - Excretory phase(8–10 mins after contrast administration) to evaluate injury to the collecting systems.

Radiological classification of renal trauma (see Figure 11.6)

- Renal injuries are graded by the American Association for the Surgery of Trauma (AAST) on the basis of depth of injury and involvement of the collecting system or vasculature.
- **Grade 1:** (80% renal injuries) a) haematuria with normal imaging studies; b) contusion; c) non-expanding subcapsular hematoma without parenchymal laceration.
- **Grade 2:** a) non-expanding perinephric haematoma confined to retroperitoneum; b) laceration <1 cm deep without involvement of collecting systems.
- **Grade 3:** laceration >1 cm deep without involvement of the collecting systems.
- **Grade 4:** a) laceration extending through cortex, medulla and collecting systems; b) injury to main renal vessels; c) segmental infarction (due to thrombosis/dissection/laceration of segmental renal artery).
- **Grade 5:** a) laceration which shatters the kidney; b) devascularization of the kidney (main renal artery laceration/thrombosis; c) avulsion of the PUJ.

Pitfalls

Ensure that an excretory phase CT is obtained whenever renal trauma is suspected or collecting system injury will be missed.

Complications after renal trauma

Complication rate ranges from 3–10%.
- **Early(<4/52):** persistent urinary extravasation, urinoma, delayed bleeding(within 1-2 weeks usually), urinary fistula, abscess, hypertension.
- **Late(>4/52):** hydronephrosis, AVF, pyelonephritis, calculus formation, delayed hypertension.

Indications for intervention

The vast majority (90–95%) of renal trauma is managed conservatively. Consider intervention for:
- Superselective embolization of bleeding vessels in massive haemorrhage.
- Embolization of pseudoaneurysm/AVF.
- Percutaneous drainage of abscess/urinoma.
- Nephrosotomy +/- antegrade ureteral stent for treatment of urethral injury/ persistent urinary leak.

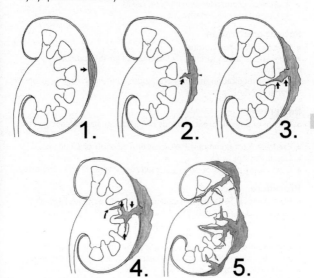

Figure 11.6 AAST grading of renal trauma.

Further reading

Kawashima, A. et al. (2001) Imaging of Renal Trauma: A Comprehensive Review. *Radiographics.* **21**: 557–74.

Renal embolization

(see 📖 Chapter 17)

Indications
- Pre-nephrectomy for large RCC.
- Trauma: Iatrogenic (e.g. post nephrostomy) or sharp/blunt renal injury.
- AML > 4 cm.
- End-stage renal disease (where surgery contra-indicated).
- Alternative to nephrectomy, e.g. where patient unfit for surgery.
- Renal artery aneurysm/arterio-venous malformation.

Contra-indications
- No absolute contra-indications.
- Relative:
  - Active/uncontrolled urinary tract sepsis.
  - Untreated coagulopathy.

Patient preparation
- Bloods: FBC/U&Es/clotting.
- Intravenous access (preferably minimum of an 18G cannula).
- Consent.
- Stop any medication that may predispose to haemorrhage (e.g. aspirin, warfarin, NSAID).

Equipment
- Choice of embolic agent depends on indication, size of feeding vessel, availability.
- Particles: most commonly PVA (polyvinyl alcohol) or Gelfoam.
- Liquid: ethanol.
- Coil: variety of coils of varying sizes, thrombogenicity and composition.

Procedure
- Medication: 1) Sedation: midazolam (1 mg boluses); 2) Analgesia: fentanyl (25 mg boluses); 3) Antibiotics: pre and post procedure according to local prescribing guidelines.
- Percutaneous access via common femoral artery.
- Cannulization of renal artery using appropriate catheter (usually 5F Cobra, sidewinder or double renal curve) and hydrophilic wire.
- Diagnostic angiogram performed to delineate anatomy.
- If main renal artery to be embolized proceed to embolization.
- If selective catheterization of branch of renal artery then proceed with 2–3F microcatheter. This can be fed through the main (e.g. Cobra) catheter over a 0.018 wire. If having difficulty make use of hydrophilic microcatheter (e.g. 'ProGreat'). Confirm position regularly by injecting contrast.

TIPS:

❶ *Balloon occlusion catheter within the renal artery can be used prior to delivery of embolic agent (e.g. absolute ethanol) thereby minimizing risk of reflux/distant embolization.*

Pitfalls

- Coil migration: ensure coil is appropriately sized for vessel. Secure catheter position before delivery.
- When injecting particle embolic agents ensure that there is no reflux into non-target territory.

Complications

- **Migration of embolic agent**: coils may dislodge and occlude peripheral vessels most commonly leg arteries. Particles and liquid agents can reflux and affect distal vasculature causing thrombosis.
- **Complications relating to angiographic technique**, e.g. renal artery dissection, groin haematoma.
- **Post-embolization syndrome:** fever, pain, leucocytosis.
- **Renal abscess.**
- **Renal failure.**
- **Incomplete embolization** (may require further attempts).

Varicocoele embolization

A varicocoele is defined as an abnormal dilatation of the pampiniform venous plexus and occurs as a result of incompetent gonadal vein valves in males. This condition manifests clinically as pain, swelling or infertility. Incidence is 5–17%. It is ten times more common on the left.

TIPS:

❶ *Rapidly enlarging or new right sided varicocoeles need further imaging to exclude retroperitoneal abnormality (e.g. kidney tumour).*

Diagnosis

Radiological diagnosis is best achieved using colour Doppler ultrasound. Look for abnormally dilated veins in the pampiniform venous plexus in the upper scrotum. Classically 2 mm has been used as the upper limit of normal for diagnosing dilated veins although some authors use 3 mm. Evaluate for reflux flow through the dilated veins on coughing or after valsalva manoeuvre.

Indications

- Symptomatic varicocoele.
- Recurrent varicocoele after previous surgery or intervention.
- Infertility (with confirmed semen abnormalities).
- Venography alone may be used to evaluate equivocal ultrasound findings.

Contraindications

- No absolute contra-indications.
- Relative:
  - Primary infertility.
  - Aberrant gonadal vasculature.
  - Untreated coagulopathy.

Patient preparation

- Bloods: FBC/U&Es/clotting.
- Intravenous access (preferably minimum of an 18G cannula).
- Consent.
- Stop any medication that may predispose to haemorrhage (e.g. aspirin, warfarin, NSAID).
- Review previous imaging to confirm diagnosis.

Equipment

Procedure

- Medication: Sedation – midazolam (1 mg boluses) may be required in the anxious patient.
- Patient positioned supine.
- Venous access via internal jugular or femoral venous approach (ultrasound guided).

TIPS:

❶ *The neck approach is favoured by the authors as this allows for easier cannulation of the renal and spermatic veins.*

- A standard 18G needle or micro-puncture kit (20–22G) can be used.
- Place a 7F sheath over a standard J wire then advance a curved catheter (e.g. Berenstein) to guide the wire through the right atrium.
- Once below the diaphragm replace standard wire with 0.035 hydrophilic wire and use this to locate the left renal vein.
- More often than not, with the catheter angled inferolaterally, the wire will lead directly into the spermatic vein.
- If this fails manoeuvre catheter into renal vein, perform venogram to identify origin of spermatic vein and manipulate wire in this region.
- Once successful follow with catheter to upper third of vein and perform venogram to a) confirm diagnosis; and b) plan the embolization site.
- Commence embolization at or above level of inguinal ring (same level as superior pubic ramus).
- Coils and microcoils are most frequently used, although detachable balloons and liquid agents can be used.
- Place multiple coils until adequate haemostasis is achieved (the upper level is usually the mid/upper third of the spermatic vein).
- Check venography is performed to confirm technical success.
- Remove catheter, wire and sheath and apply manual compression for 3–5minutes.
- Technical success rate >90%.

Pitfalls

- Venous spasm is fairly common but responds poorly to vasodilators (e.g. glyceryl trinitrate).
- Observe carefully for venous collaterals and for optimum results place coils at level of collateral origin.
- Occasionally embolization of iliac vein tributaries may be required.

Complications

- Recurrence is seen in 10%, and the most common causes include missed collateral veins, recanalization of occluded segments and poorly positioned coils.
- Migration of embolic material is rarely reported.
- Testicular thrombophlebitis.
- Complications relating to the vascular access are rare but include haematoma, pneumothorax, and cellulitis.

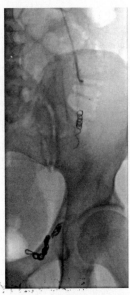

Figure 11.7 Varicocele embolization. Coils deployed at level of the inguinal ring. Second set of coils deployed at mid-point of testicular vein to treat small collateral veins.

Further reading

Kessel, D. and Robertson, I. (2005) *Interventional Radiology: A Survival Guide*. Elsevier.

http://www.emedicine.com/radio/topic739.htm.

Haemodialysis fistula

Haemodialysis fistula

Fistula's require >500 mls of flow per minute for optimum function.

Native AVF's: usually start at the wrist in the non dominant hand, i.e. radio-cephalic (Brescia-Cimino), gradually progressing proximally, i.e. brachio-basilic , axillary, etc.

- Long lasting (revision rate of only 15% year).
- Reliable.
- Low infection.
- Low thrombosis.
- Generally perform better than grafts with much better long term patency.

Arteiovenous grafts: These are much more popular in the USA than in the Europe, however these are used when both the upper limbs' native veins are exhausted, utilizing either upper limbs or groins.

- Grafts have the advantage that they can be used almost immediately while AVF's require several weeks/months for maturation.

Disadvantages of grafts:

- Higher thrombosis.
- Higher infection.
- Higher rate of revision or re-intervention (80% per year).

Xenografts, i.e. Bovine ureter synergrafts: used when all veins used and as an alternative to dacron grafts. These behave more like AV grafts although experience with these is limited.

There is a high incidence of complications, in particular thrombosis. It is estimated that arteriovenous fistula (AVF) have an incidence of 0.2 per patient/year and for grafts 0.8–1 per patient/year. Prospective surveillance (Table 12.1) combined with prophylactic surgery or PTA improves cumulative patency up to 70%.

Monitoring of venous pressure, flow or both combined with PTA reduces the incidence of thrombosis in grafts to <0.5 events per patient/year.

Surveillance

Table 12.1 Methods of surveillance for arteriovenous fistula (AVF)

Clinical evaluation
Physical evaluation
Bleeding time
Recirculation
Static access pressure
Arterial intra-access pressure
Venous intra-access pressure
Dynamic venous pressure
Blood flow measurement
Doppler ultrasound
Thermal dilution

Common problems

- Steal: large fistulas or distal disease result in ischemia to the distal limb. High flow fistulas usually require surgical banding or may require closure.
- Stenosis: depending on the site will result in oedema, prolonged bleeding (outflow venous stenosis) or inadequate dialysis (arterial/anastomotic) and both result in occlusion.
- Failure to mature: usually due to arterial disease or large accessory veins.
- Oedema: this is usually due to venous obstruction or due to high flow.
- Aneurysm: extremely common and usually requires no therapy. Occasionally false aneurysms develop which may require treatment either with thrombin injection or stenting.

Clinical evaluation

Swelling in the access arm and multiple subcutaneous collateral veins at the neck, shoulder, and upper chest are suggestive of central vein stenosis. Not all central vein stenoses cause these signs.

Fistula assessment

- The anastomosis is assessed by examination of the thrill, which is an indicator of flow, the pulse, an indicator of downstream resistance, and the bruit. The thrill and the bruit are prominent near the anastomosis and are present in systole and early diastole (continuous).
- A stenosis reduces the strength of the thrill. If away from the anastomosis, the thrill and bruit occur only in systole. A forceful, 'water-hammer' pulse, suggests a stenosis.
- The thrill and bruit gradually diminish away from the anastomosis. Increase in the thrill or a new thrill downstream suggests a stenosis. The pulse becomes hard in the presence of a body stenosis.
- Elevation of the arm above the level of the heart normally collapses the pulse. The segment upstream from a stenosis does not collapse but the downstream segment does collapse.
- Accessory veins (single or multiple) limit the maturation of the AV fistulas. An accessory vein <a quarter the diameter of the main vessel is unlikely to be significant. When the fistula is occluded proximally, the thrill at the fistula disappears. Palpation of the main vein below the site of occlusion will reveal a thrill at the site of the accessory vein.
- Pulse augmentation. The AVF is occluded proximally and with the other hand the pulse palpated next to the anastomosis. The pulse should become hyperpulsatile. If not, indicative of arterial, anastomotic, or juxta-anastomotic stenosis.

Surveillance assessment of fistula indicative of a significant stenoses of >50% or presence of accessory veins. i.e:

- Difficulty during cannulation.
- Frequent withdrawal of clots.
- Increased venous pressures.
- Decreased flow rates at dialysis (<500–600 mL/minute in autogenous AVF's and <600–800 mL/minute for grafts); or
- Reduction of 20–25% compared to previous measurements.

- Increase in the ratio of aIAP (arterial Intra-access Pressure)/vIAP (venous Intra-Access Pressure) by 0.2 units over time is also indication for evaluation (Table 12.2).
- Following clinical evaluation as shown above.

Table 12.2 Criteria for referring patient for angiography/intervention using intra-access pressure in AVF

Stenoses degree	vIAP/MAP	aIAP/MAP
<50%	0.13 to 0.43	0.08 to 0.34
>50% in:		
Venous outflow segment	≥ 0.44	or 0.35
Mid-segment	≥ 0.44	and <0.35+ clinical signs
Arterial inflow segment	< 0.13 + clinical signs	

Pressures are normalized for mean arterial pressure at the arterial puncture site (aIAP) and at the venous puncture site (vIAP).

Direct imaging is performed when these surveillance techniques suggest a significant stenosis.

- Color Doppler ultrasonography (Figure 12.1) is a readily available, inexpensive, and non-invasive. However, it is operator dependant, unable to detect central obstruction and gives no angiographic map, for surgery or percutaneous therapy.
- Digital subtraction angiography (DSA) is the gold standard for the evaluation of access patency but is invasive.
- Contrast-enhanced magnetic resonance angiography (CE-MRA) and Computer tomography angiography (CTA) can also be used for evaluation fistulas and grafts.

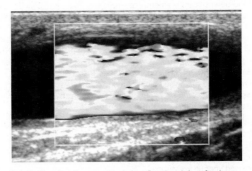

Figure 12.1 Duplex showing normal turbulent flow in a dialysis fistula.

PTA

Percutaneous transluminal angioplasty (Figure 12.2) has become a standard treatment for the correction of stenosis in AVF and AV graft.

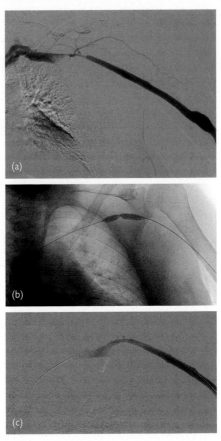

Figure 12.2 (a) Cephalic arch stenosis in a brachio-cephalic fistula. (b) Venoplasty. (c) Post venoplasty.

Advantages over surgical procedure
- It is an outpatient procedure.
- It does not prohibit the immediate use of access for dialysis.
- It has minimal to no blood loss; hospitalization is avoided; and rarely is there discomfort to the patient.

- The only disadvantage is that there are some lesions that do not respond to treatment and the results obtained are not permanent.

The K/DOQI panel states that waiting for graft thrombosis before intervention leads to increased graft failure. The correction of a subcritical (50–70%) stenosis by PTA is more likely to be successful than correction of a critical (90–98%) fibrotic stenosis. The need for re-intervention is high.

- Technical success is high: 79–94%
- Primary patency 6 months   >60%
- Primary patency 12 months   >35%
- Complications   4–5%

TIPS:

- Rupture: Try simple prolonged balloon tamponade or compression over the rupture as the fistulas are very superficial or a combination of the two. Bare stenting may close the rupture if the above fails or stentgraft (much more expensive and larger sheath size).
- False aneurysm, very rarely necessary to treat, try thrombin if narrow neck with or without balloon or short covered stent (Figure 12.3).
- Puncture site haematoma: Prevention using a purse string suture around the puncture site prior to removal of the sheath will reduce this (with or without woggle modification) (Figure 12.4).
- Emboli: Often clot in the fistula, particularly in the aneurysmal segments, but emboli to the lungs are usually small and of no sequelae.

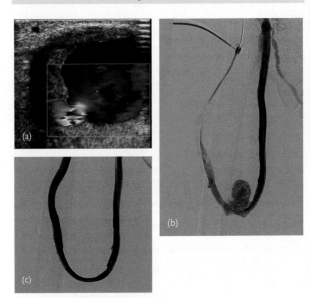

Figure 12.3 (a) Duplex showing large false aneurysm. (b) Fistulogram confirming aneurysm. (c) Post-stentgrafting.

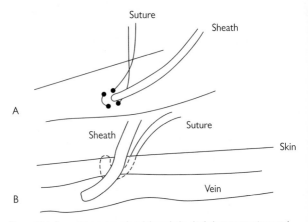

Figure 12.4 Purse string suture placed through the skin/subcutaneous tissue and through the upper wall of the vessel around the sheath. The two ends are then tied in a knot as the sheath is withdrawn or can be held in place by placing a little cuff held there by a clip (woggle technique).

Indications for intervention

- Stenoses >50%, Most are at the venous anastomosis and needling sites. Central stenosis usually relate to previous central lines.
- Occlusion.
- Presence of accessory veins.

Contra-indications for intervention

- Local sepsis.
- Severe derangement of clotting parameters.

Equipment

- Sheath 4–12F (size depends on balloons/devices used).
- Standard balloons.
- Additional equipment: high pressure balloons/cutting balloons.
- Stents/Stengrafts: size range 6–14 mm.
- Antiplatelet agents: some evidence to support using antiplatelet agents.
- Heparin.
- Routinely administered at the time of angioplasty (PTA), but no evidence of improved outcomes to angioplasty without heparin.

Technique

- Always use a sheath.
- Easiest from the venous part of the fistula itself, may be necessary or to use the femoral, subclavian, or jugular vein approach for venous stenosis. Femoral or brachial arterial approach for upstream arterial or peri anastomotic lesions. The technique for venoplasty is identical to that for angioplasty in arteries (see 🕮 Chapter 5).
- Venous strictures: often highly fibrotic and high pressure balloons or cuttings balloons may be required (Figure 12.5).
- Cutting balloons should not be used immediately after standard balloon venoplasty as there is an increased risk of rupture. Should be used first to create the dissection plane and then the standard balloon to get the vein to the desired size. Used most commonly for failed venoplasty . Some advocate this for primary use to reduce the barotrauma during venoplasty.

TIPS:

Options for treating occlusions include:
- Standard catheter/guidewire techniques.
- Sharp recanalization (Figure 12.6) using the stiff end of a guidewire, i.e. Terumo and curved catheter to dissect through or Calapinto needle.
- Use collaterals, some can be very large and develop stenosis which may respond to angioplasty.

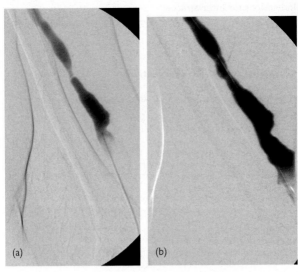

Figure 12.5 (a) Pre-cutting balloon venoplasty. (b) Post-cutting balloon venoplasty.

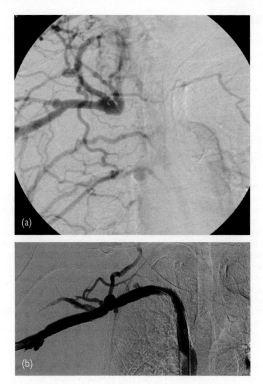

Figure 12.6 (a) Chronic occusion of brachiocephalic vein and SVC pre sharp recanalization using a 5F Cobra catheter and the stiff end of a Terumo wire to dissect through the SVC. (b) Post sharp recanalization and stenting.

Stenting

Indications

- Uncontrolled rupture.
- Elastic recoil.
- Repeated recurrence.
- PTA plus primary stent.

Stents function as an endoskeleton and provide supportive expansion to diseased vessels. Results with newer bare metal stents and drug-eluting stents appear promising. Improvement in graft survival (88% at 6 months and 86% at 12 months) over conventional surgical or angioplasty techniques.

Avoid: At venous junctions, dialysis puncture sites or small veins <5 mm and in the presence of sepsis.

Thrombosed grafts

Duplex is helpful is gauging the extent of the occlusion. For grafts the thrombus is often limited to the graft itself. There are several techniques for clearing these:

- Thrombolytic agents including the newer drugs such as tenecteplase. Used either on their own or in combination with mechanical thrombectomy. Additional PTA or surgery will almost certainly be required, to treat the underlying stenosis.
- Immediate success rate is higher in grafts (99% v. 94% for forearm grafts and fistulas), the primary patency rates are higher for AVFs compared to grafts (49% v. 14%).
- One year secondary patency rates are 80% and 50% respectively for forearm and for upper arm AVFs.
- Complications: Primarily haemorrhagic 7–9%
- Technique: see below.

Thrombolysis

- Be aware of contraindication and risks (see 📖 Chapter 6).
- Patients should be closely observed, ideally in a HDU.
- For AV fistulas it is often possible to puncture above the thrombus aiming for the anastomosis and place a multiside hole catheter as close to the anastomosis as possible (Figure 12.7). For extensive thrombus and grafts a criss-cross technique whereby a puncture 10–15 cm from the arterial anastomosis directed towards the anastomosis and another puncture 5 cm distal to the anastomosis towards the central veins is made. So that two 4–5F multisided hole catheters are placed crossing each other and simultaneous thrombolysis can then be performed.
- The thrombus is then laced with 4–5 mg of rTPA and then an infusion commenced at 0.5–1 mg rTPA per hour. There is usually rapid clearance of thrombus and regular catheter venography should be performed with catheter repositioning to optimize rTPA infusion into the thrombus. There may be a small residual clot or plug particularly at the anastomosis which can usually be angioplastied while dealing with the underlying stenosis.

Mechanical lysis

- Using the above puncture technique, a mechanical device can be subsitituted. These have the advantage of speed and potentially lower complications. These devices include fragmentation devices such as the
- Teratola (Figure 12.8);
- Oasis;
- Amplatzer
- Rotarex; (Figure 12.9);

or rheolytic devices:

- Angiojet;
- Hyrolyser;

or both fragmentation and lysis:

- Trellis (Figure 12.10).

The greatest experience is with the Teratola device. This is a 7F, over the wire (0.25) rotating basket, which fragments clot (Figures 12.10a-c) . However, with this device caution is needed in small veins (not <6 mm diameter) and should be avoided with patients with stents (Figure 12.10d)

- Technical Success 87–95%.
- Clinical success 79–89%.
- 6 month primary patency 38–60%.
- Complications 4–9%.

Clot aspiration: Using a 6–8F guiding catheter, thrombus can be directly aspirated from the AVF or graft. This can be very successful and quick in a limited, acute soft clot.

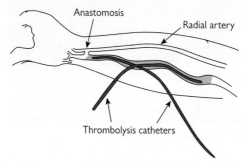

Figure 12.7 Criss cross technique for thrombolysis. Multi-sidehole cathetes are introduced either using a sheath or bare from the venous and arterial ends of the fistula. Then lysis agents are infused simultaneously to clear the thrombus.

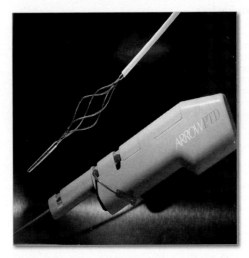

Figure 12.8 Teratola fragmentation device.

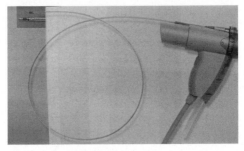

Figure 12.9 Rotarex fragmentation device.

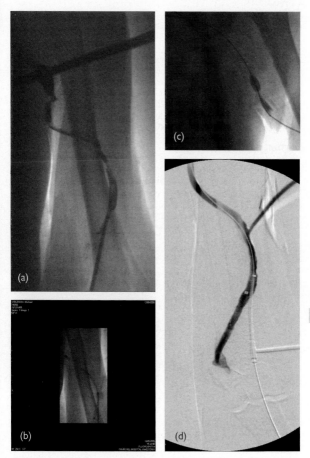

Figure 12.10 Sequence of images (a-d) showing clearing of thrombosed graft using a Teratola device to macerate clot into small particles which are taken up by the lungs and venoplasty of outflow stenosis.

Failure of maturation

- Inflow stenosis, i.e. arterial or juxta-anastomotic:
  - Angioplasty as above.
- Accessory veins:
  - Usually accessory veins require surgical ligation, however an alternative would be to embolize large collaterals using coils to help develop the main vein.
- Small veins:
  - Despite waiting several months some veins don't enlarge and these can be encouraged to develop by gradual dilatation using an increasing size of balloon over a period of several weeks.

Further reading

Bay W.H., Henry M.L., Lazarus J.M., Lew N.L., Ling J. and Lowrie E.G. (1998) Predicting hemodialysis access failure with color flow. Doppler ultrasound. *Am J Nephrol.* **18**: 296–304.

Besarab A., Sullivan K.L., Ross R.P. and Morritz M.J. (1995). Utility of intra-access pressure monitoring in detecting and correcting venous outlet stenoses prior to thrombosis. *Kidney Int.* **47**: 1364–73.

Kanterman R.Y., Vesely T.M., Pilgram T.K., Guy B.W., Windus D.W. and Picus D. (1995) Dialysis access grafts: anatomic location of venous stenosis and results of angioplasty. *Radiology* **195**: 135–9.

NKF-K/DOQI clinical practice guidelines for vascular access: Update 2000. *Am J Kidney Dis.* 2001; **37**: S137–S181.

Tordoir J.H.M., Van Der Sande F.M. and De Hann M.W. (2004) Current topics on vascular access for Haemodialysis. *Minerva Urol Nefrol.* **56**: 223–35.

Hepatobiliary intervention

PTC, biliary drainage and stenting – PTC vs ERCP

PTC is now rarely required for diagnostic purposes, as it has been replaced by non invasive techniques such as US, MRI/MRCP, and CT.

It remains an important method for accessing the biliary tract for drainage and dilatation/stenting of strictures.

PTC and ERCP are complementary techniques, and the approach used will depend on local expertise. However, in general terms ERCP is the preferred technique for the management of bile duct stones and bile duct strictures, particularly in the ducts below the hilum.

A percutaneous approach is often preferred for strictures involving the hilum, where insertion of bilateral stents may be required.

Percutaneous biliary drainage and stenting

(see 📖 Chapter 10)

Indications
- Palliation of obstructive jaundice due to:
- Malignant biliary stricture.
- Benign biliary stricture.
- Treatment of cholangitis ± CBD stones (where ERCP fails or is not possible).

Contraindications
- Deranged clotting (this should be corrected).

Note: Ascites is not an absolute contraindication, but if large in volume then consider draining this first.

Technique
- Obtain informed consent.
- Check the platelet count and the clotting and correct any abnormalities.
- Give antibiotics (check local policy).
- Conscious sedation and local anaesthesia are usually administered, but there are other options, e.g. nerve blocks and general anaesthesia may be required on occasion.
- Decide on the approach – the right sided ducts may be punctured using either fluoroscopy or ultrasound, the left require ultrasound guidance.
- For the right sided ducts the usual approach is through the intercostal space, just above the tenth rib, in the mid axillary line.
- Infiltrate with local anaesthetic to liver capsule.
- Propriety kits which contain a Chiba needle, 0.018 wire, and sheath/dilator are useful
- The Chiba needle (22G) is inserted, and if using fluoroscopy it should be advanced towards the xiphisternum until the level of the transverse process of the vertebral body is reached (Figure 13.1).

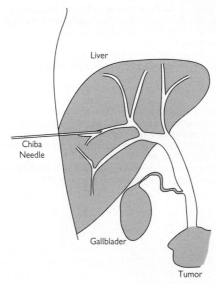

Figure 13.1 Transverse pass through the liver in approximately the mid-axillary line, parallel to the table top. The Chiba needle is gradually withdrawn slowly until bile is aspirated with a tube and syringe or alternatively contrast is injected intermittently to check if a duct has been entered.

- The central stylet is withdrawn and contrast is slowly injected as the needle is withdrawn, until a duct is entered. This will be recognized as a characteristic 'swirling' effect as the contrast mixes with bile. When the needle tip is within a vessel, the contrast flows away, usually this will be either towards the IVC (hepatic vein) or towards the periphery of the liver (portal vein).
- If a duct is not entered then the needle position is maintained within the liver capsule and a slightly different approach is taken, angling cranially/caudally until a duct is punctured.
- If the duct puncture is central and the stricture involves the hilum, it may be necessary to subsequently puncture a more peripheral duct, once these have been opacified with contrast.
- In these circumstances, many operators would elect to perform the initial puncture under US guidance to select a peripheral duct initially.

TIPS:

Having opacified the peripheral biliary tree. For the second puncture the parallax technique is used. By angling the C arm LAO or RAO to it is possible to assess if the needle is passing in front or behind the duct and the needle orientated accordingly (see Figure 13.2).

- Once in the duct, the 0.018 guidewire may be advanced towards the CBD. The needle is removed and the sheath/dilator inserted.
- The 0.018 wire and dilator are removed and an 0.035 Amplatz wire may now be inserted.
- It will now be possible to insert a larger, e.g. 6–8F sheath. Those with radio-opaque markers are useful, particularly when stent insertion is planned.
- At this stage, more contrast may be injected to demonstrate, e.g. the stricture, and if biliary drainage is all that is required or planned then an external biliary drain (pigtail catheter) can be placed.
- However it is often possible to manipulate a wire through the stricture and into the duodenum. This may be achieved with a variety of catheters (e.g. Cobra, or biliary manipulation catheter) and often requires use of a hydrophilic wire.
- Once through into duodenum the wire should be exchanged for an Amplatz and passed along the duodenal loop to D3/4.

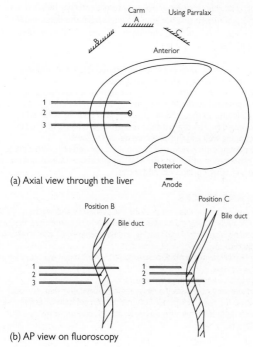

(a) Axial view through the liver

(b) AP view on fluoroscopy

Figure 13.2 By angling the C arm from AP (A) to RAO (B) and LAO (C) it is possible to assess if the needle is anterior or posterior by how it moves in relation go the duct (b).

It is then possible to insert either an 'internal/external' biliary drain (which has sufficient side holes to drain bile from the ducts above the stricture across into the duodenum) (Figure 13.3a) or a stent (Figure 13.3b).

- If a metal stent is inserted it can be balloon dilated to improve expansion in particularly tight strictures.
- Once a stent has been inserted it is common for an operator to leave some external access (e.g. a pigtail drain) in situ within the ducts above the stricture, so that a check cholangiogram can be obtained the following day. The drain is then removed, assuming that the stent is functioning well and the ducts are decompressed.
- The patient is then returned to the ward for bed rest with a protocol for observation of T, P and BP. The complications to look out for are bleeding, biliary peritonitis, and sepsis.

TIPS AND TRICKS:
- Be aware that bile can track along the catheters and wires, particularly during exchanges, and cause biliary peritonitis. Perform exchanges smoothly and quickly and be prepared to give analgesia as required.
- Particularly with 'central' punctures, the track may well cross fairly large vessels.
  These may be identified when removing your sheath over a guidewire and injecting contrast. If a large vessel is identified then consider embolizing the track peripheral to this with gelfoam or coils.
  Some routinely embolize the track to reduce symptoms due to biliary leak.

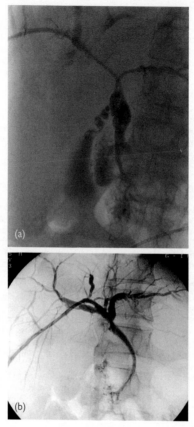

Figure 13.3 (a) Patient with hilar obstruction with bilateral access and drains. (b) Patient with a distal obstruction due to pancreatic carcinoma. A Nitis biliary stent (Pyramed UK) has been placed with a 8F drain left in situ.

Stents

- Plastic stents are much cheaper than metal stents, but they do not last as long as they block more quickly.
- Plastic stents that extend through the ampulla can be removed fairly readily endoscopically, whereas most metal stents cannot be removed.
- Metal stents usually require only a 6–7F percutaneous access track and then expand up to 10 mm.
- Uncovered metal stents may allow improved drainage at sites where ducts branch, e.g. at the hilum.
- A single stent will suffice for strictures in the lower and middle third of the bile duct, and in hilar disease where one lobe has atrophied significantly.
- Bilateral (i.e. right and left duct) stents may have advantages, giving improved drainage in strictures involving the main right and left hepatic ducts.
- There are now also T or Y configured stents to allow simultaneous draingae of both duct systems (Figure 13.4).
- The aim of a palliative biliary stent is to relieve jaundice and pruritis, and this can usually be achieved by draining a relatively small proportion of the liver (approximately one sixth). However, opacifying ducts with contrast and then not draining them increases the risk of infection. Therefore it is worth studying the images (CT, MRCP) beforehand and planning your approach with this in mind.

Note on benign strictures

- These may be inflammatory (e.g. PSC) or post surgical (e.g. following transplant/choledocho-jejunostomy).
- They are difficult to treat and often require repeated procedures.
- Treatment options include repeated inflations with high pressure balloons ± plastic stent insertion.
- Retrievable metal stents have been introduced for this condition, and their value is currently being evaluated.
- Some surgeons leave a Roux loop for access adhered to the anterior abdominal wall, and there may be staples visible at fluoroscopy to help guide your puncture into this loop.

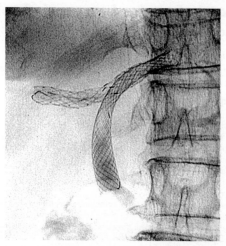

Figure 13.4 Nitis T stent configuration to drain both left and right ducts. © Pyramed.

Removal of retained stones via T-tube track

Indications
Retained stones, demonstrated on a T-tube cholangiogram, where ERCP is not possible.

Technique
- Ideally the T-tube should be >12F and stones <10 mm.
- It is left in situ for four weeks for the track to mature.
- It may be necessary to dilate the tract gradually up to 24+F over one or two sessions so as not to rupture the tract. This can be done with a balloon or Teflon dilaters.
- Antibiotic cover.
- Patient supine, cholangiogram obtained and then T-tube slowly removed.
- A steerable catheter/wire basket combination is manipulated along the track and into the bile duct, with its tip adjacent to the stone.
- The basket is opened, engaging (capturing) the stone, and the whole ensemble is slowly removed along the track.
- Larger stones may require fragmentation with a lithotripser, and multiple stones/fragments will require multiple passes.
- Be prepared for several visits to clear the ducts of all stones and fragments leaving a large drain each time.
- In practice this technique is rarely required these days, as stones can usually be removed endoscopically or laparoscopically.

Cholecystostomy

(see 📖 Chapter 19)

Percutaneous drainage of the gall bladder may be required in the following circumstances:

- Gallbladder empyema.
- Acute cholecystitis not settling after 48 hrs conservative treatment.
- Investigation of unexplained sepsis in critically ill patients.

The principles of percutaneous drainage are covered elsewhere. Points pertinent to gall bladder drainage are:

- The approach – you will often read that a transhepatic approach is best. This may be true but it is not always easy/possible in an enlarged inflamed gall bladder which has become adherent to the anterior abdominal wall. In this instance a transperitoneal approach is often more practical. T fasteners may be helpful in this situation (see 📖 pg. 290) to anchor the GB.
- A self retaining pigtail catheter is useful, remembering that as the gallbladder decompresses it will tend to shrink away from the catheter and dislodgement is a risk (this is not a problem with the transhepatic approach).
- A cholecystogram should be obtained prior to removing the catheter (which is often left in situ for 2 weeks) to check that the cystic duct is now patent and that there is free flow into duodenum (to avoid biliary fistula and/or recurrent symptoms).
- Occasionally this technique can be used as an alternative to PTC for access for drainage and stenting and gallstone removal.

Endoscopic retrograde cholangiopancreatography (ERCP)

ERCP is now rarely required as a diagnostic tool, as it has been replaced by non-invasive imaging methods such as US, CT, and MRI/MRCP. It remains an important and widely used technique for the treatment of biliary disorders, and is usually the procedure of choice for treating bile duct stones and CBD strictures.

A detailed account of the procedure is beyond the scope of this book, and a brief outline is given below.

Conditions managed by ERCP
- Bile duct stones.
- Malignant biliary strictures
- Benign biliary strictures.
- Biliary leaks (e.g. following surgery or trauma).
- Sphincter of Oddi disorder (SOD).
- Pancreatic disorders.

Advantages of ERCP
- Direct visualization and biopsy of duodenum and ampulla.
- Stones can be removed and stents inserted without traversing liver.

Disadvantages
- Not possible after some types of surgery or with duodenal (D1/2) obstruction.
- Complications (see below).
- Mortality 0.1–1%.

Complications
- Pancreatitis.
- Haemorrhage.
- Cholangitis.
- Perforation.

Pancreatic intervention

Stents for strictures, e.g. pancreatic pseudocyst communication with the duct, pancreatic ascites.

Further reading

Cotton, P.B., Williams, C.B., Sleisenger, M.H. *Practical Gastrointestinal Endoscopy : The Fundamentals* 5th Edn, Blackwell Scientific Publications.

Endoscopic ultrasound (EUS)

The proximity of the luminal GI tract to the mediastinum, pancreas, hepato-biliary system, and adrenal glands and the development of ech-oendoscopes with 3.2 and 3.8 mm working channels, has lead to the development of a number of EUS guided interventional procedures.

The details are beyond the scope of this book, but the interventional radiologist should at least be aware of availability of this technique for the following:

- Lymph node staging, e.g. for upper GI, pancreatic and lung cancers.
- Fine needle aspiration and/or biopsy of submucosal GI tumours, adrenal lesions and pancreatic masses.
- Pseudocyst drainage.
- Drainage of mediastinal collections.
- Coeliac plexus block (carcinoma pancreas, chronic pancreatitis).

This is an evolving technology and further developments are likely in the near future, e.g. targeted tumour therapy.

Further reading

Hawes, R., Fockens, P. (2006) *Endosonography*, Saunders. Elsevier.

Gastro-intestinal intervention

Oesophageal stenting

Indications
- Malignant oesophageal stricture – either for palliation or to improve nutrition prior to treatment.
- Extrinsic compression from mediastinal tumour.
- Fistula between oesophagus and tracheal/bronchus.
- Oesophageal perforation.
- Malignant anastomotic leak/recurrent tumour.
- Benign strictures – refractory to balloon dilatation (consider retrievable stent).

Contraindications
- No absolute contraindications.
- Relative contraindications:
  - Coagulopathy.
  - Patient unfit for conscious sedation.
  - Recent high dose chemotherapy/radiotherapy.
  - Obstructed stomach/small bowel.
  - Severe tracheal compression.
  - High strictures close to vocal cords.

Types of stents available
- All self expanding.
- Generally metal with plastic covering.
- 16–18F delivery system.
- Typically 16–24 mm expanded diameter.
- Anti reflux valve option.
- Retrievable option.

Uncovered stents
- Reduced risk of migration.
- Increased risk of blockage due to tumour in-growth.
- May be useful in extrinsic compression, hugely dilated oesophagus, gastric pull-through.

Covered stents
- Improved designs with proximal ± distal flowing, partial covering and covering on inside of stent have reduced the risk of migration.
- Now first choice in most situations.

Anti-reflux valve stents
Reduce acid reflux post stent insertion across gastro-oesophageal junction.

Retrievable stents
Can be removed endoscopically for a limited period (see manufacturer's recommendations for individual stents), or left in permanently. They are useful in the following circumstances:
- Benign strictures – for a limited time, e.g. 6–8 weeks, to give a prolonged dilatation.
- Where tolerance of stent is questionable – e.g. in high strictures.

- As a bridge to surgery, allowing improved nutrition in the pre-operative period.
- To allow a fistula/perforation to seal.

Technique

- Perform a preliminary contrast swallow to define site and length of stricture.
- Patient usually in lateral position.
- Anaesthetic (xylocaine) throat spray and conscious sedation with P, BP and O_2 monitoring.
- Per oral catheter – e.g. biliary manipulation catheter (BMC), or multi-purpose catheter, into oesophagus.
- Contrast injected to delineate stricture.
- Stiff guidewire (Amplatz) passed across stricture and into gastric antrum/D1 (use hydrophilic wire to cross stricture initially if necessary and then exchange).
- Stent delivery device passed over guidewire and across stricture.
- Markers on the stent/delivery system are visible with fluoroscopy allowing accurate placement of device across stricture.
- Stent deployed, generally by pulling back the outer sheath, under fluoroscopic guidance, and with slightly more stent above than below stricture.
- A follow-up swallow, e.g. at 24 hours will confirm stent position and function (Figure 14.1).

TIPS/CAUTION:

- Approximately 60% of the stent should be above the stricture to reduce risk of migration.
- Anti-reflux valves useful for lesions requiring stents to cross the GOJ (redcue need for proton pump inhibitors) but may obstruct more easily.
- Beware proximal lesions near cricopharangeus (C6/7). Stents which don't shorten or are retrievable may be better for these lesions.
- Don't use large Flamingo stents for mid or proimal oesophageal lesions (risk of aortic fistula).

Aftercare

- Start with oral fluids.
- Progress to low residue diet.
- Provide patients with dietary advice sheet, i.e.:
  - Avoid lumps of food and chew well.
  - Take plenty of fluid with meals.
  - Fizzy drinks can be helpful.
  - Treat any reflux symptoms with a protein pump inhibitor.
  - Stay upright for 1 hour after meals (particularly for GOJ stents).

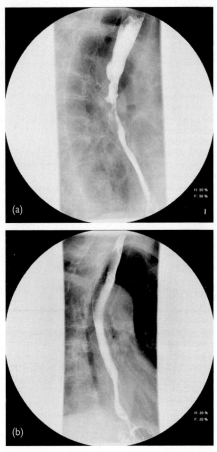

Figure 14.1 (a) Pre-stent swallow shows tight stricture at the junction of the middle and lower third of the oesophagus. (b) Post-stent swallow shows good flow of barium.

Benign strictures

Caution required – there will be initial clinical relief of symptoms but a recurrent dysphagia rate of almost 100%, due to tissue hyperplasia blocking the stent, if left in situ long term.

If stenting is required, consider a retrievable option.

Complications

- Haemorrhage 3–8%.
- Prolonged chest pain 14%.
- Migration 0–10%.
- Tumour in-growth:
  - uncovered 17–36%.
  - covered 0–1%.
- Perforation 2–3%.
- Death 0–1.4%.

Gastric/gastroduodenal stents

Indications
- Linitus plastica – stents are not very helpful in the author's experience.
- Gastric outflow/proximal duodenal obstruction, e.g. due to carcinoma of pancreas – can provide useful palliation.

Technique
- Can be fluoroscopic, endoscopic or a combination of the two.
- Pass a stiff (e.g. Amplatz) wire through to DJ flexure if possible, with insertion technique otherwise similar to that of oesophageal stenting.

Jejunal stents

Indications

Stricture due to inoperable tumour.

Technique

- May be possible with oral technique but difficult.
- Create gastrostomy (see 📖 pg. 290).
- Dilate tract and place 10F sheath.
- Cross pylorus into duodenum and across stricture using a combination of curved catheters (Cobra/BMC, etc.) and soft wires (Bentson). Hydrophilic wires are useful but gastric acid rapidly damages the coating and wires become sticky, so have to be quick.
- Exchange for stiff wire (Amplatz) and place stent (wall stent or Nitis).
- Fix sheath for temporary venting and access. A temporary catheter can also be left across the lesion.
- Alternatively, a direct puncture into the Jejunum just proximal to the obstruction can be peformed (see section on Gastrostomy) and this used to place a stent as above (Figure 14.2).

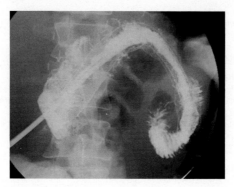

Figure 14.2 Two jejunal self expanding wallstents have been placed directly through direct jejunal access with good expansion and drainage.

References/Further reading

Sabharwal, T., Morales, J.P., Irani, A.A. (2005) C.V.I.R. **28**(3): 284–8.

Kessel, D., Robertson, I. (2005) *Interventional Radiology – A Survival Guide*, Elsevier (Churchill Livingstone)

Adam, A. Dondelinger, R.F., Mueller, P.R. (eds) (2004) *Interventional Radiology in Cancer*, Springer-Verlag.

Radiologically placed gastrostomy (RIG) or percutaneously placed gastrostomy (PIG)

The former is quicker and easier to perform. The latter has much better indwell times.

Indications
Enteral feeding but inability to swallow, i.e tumour, neurological damage.

Preparation
- Clotting:
- IV Access.
- Ideally NG tube in place.
- Barium down NG tube 24 hours before if possible.
- Single dose of antibiotic, i.e. ciprofloxacin.

Equipment
- 10 ml 1% lidocaine.
- 18 gauge needle.
- T fastners (Appendix).
- Stiff wire, i.e. Amplatz stiff.
- Dilaters 6–12F.
- >12F Peel away sheath.
- Replacement Balloon PEG or self retaining catheter.

Technique
- Check position of liver with US.
- Insufflate stomach through NG tube to distend stomach and bring below rib cage, liver, and colon.
- Puncture site over stomach should be mid way between lesser and greater curve to avoid vessels.
- Infiltrate 10 mls Lidocaine over 2 cm area over intended site.
- For gastrostomy angle towards fundus for gastrojejunostomy towards duodenum (Figure 14.3).
- Introduce T fastener needle and check position either by aspiration of air or instill tiny amount of contrast (tricky with the thread in the way)
- Place at least one T fastener as shown (Figure 14.4) some place 2–4.
- Pull stomach forward and anchor by either stiching or with the attached needle to the skin (Figure 14.5), using the clip on the suture (Harpon T fastner – Figure 14.6) or simply pull on suture.
- Introduce 18 gauge seldinger into the stomach and check position as above.
- Introduce stiff wire and dilate to appropriate size (Figure 14.7).
- Over the wire peel away sheath.
- Introduce PEG/Tube through the peelway (Figure 14.8). More secure if done over the wire.
- Inflate balloon on PEG and pull snugly to anchor in place.

TIPS:
- Introduce the guide wire through the second or third T fastener needle to reduce punctures before anchoring T fastener.
- Many need buscopan if the stomach is peristalsing and pushing air into small bowel.

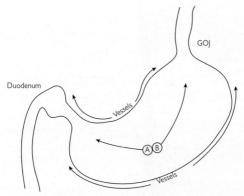

Figure 14.3 Puncture site A for gastro-jejunostomy and B for standard gastrostomy.

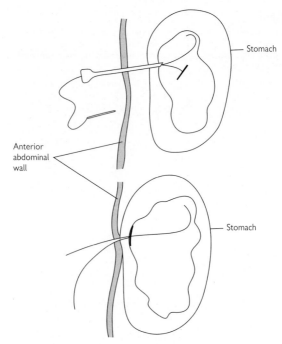

Figure 14.4 Introduction of T fasteners.

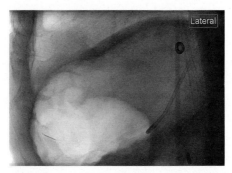

Figure 14.5 Lateral view showing anchoring of the stomach with single T fasteners.

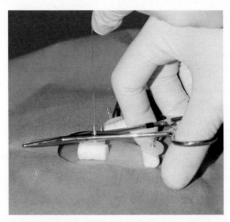

Figure 14.6 Fixing the clip on the suture using the Harpon T fasteners.

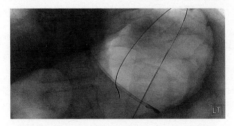

Figure 14.7 Insertion of a a guidewire through the same needle as a T fasteners.

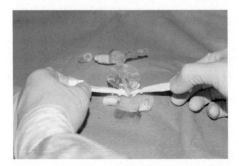

Figure 14.8 Peel away sheath being peeled off following inflation of replacement PEG balloon. © Pyramed.

PIG

This is to place a standard endoscopic type gastrostomy with a phlange, which has much better indwell time. It needs additional equipment:
- Curved catheter, i.e. BMC, Cobra, headhunter, etc.
- 7F bright tip sheath.
- Terumo Wire and long 260 cm standard wire.
- Push type Gastrostomy and adapter.

Technique

Initial technique for access identical to RIG:
- Over the stiff wire place 7F sheath.
- Use curved catheter to access GOJ.
- Pass long wire up to the mouth. Assistant grasps the end and a long catheter passed out of the mouth.
- The threads which come with the gastrostomy can sometimes be passed through the catheter and tied to the loop on the gastromy and pulled through. Sometimes a snare is required if threads won't pass. Some gastrostomy catheters will pass over the wire.
- The gastrostomy end is retrieved from the abdominal wall and pulled out until the phalange is snug, the end cut, and the adapter fixed to the end and anchored to the wall.

TIPS:
- When puncturing the stomach may need to go a little lower and laterally to get a good angle to go for the GOJ.
- Angling the tube is helpful in seeing where the NG tube enters the stomach.
- If great difficulty in accessing GOJ, snare the NG tube or wire from the NG tube and gently pull back the NG to get the catheters up the oesophagus.

Aftercare
- Erect CXR next day to exclude large pneumoperitoneum.
- Then commence water at approximately 50 ml/hr. If ok commence feeding.
- Remove T fasteners after approximately 1 week.

Technical success >95%
Complications   <5% (Peritonitis, visceral puncture, bleeding)

If the tube falls out after a week and/or the T fastners are still in, it is usually possible just to push it back. If <1 week, no T fastners and no tract then may need to start from the beginning.

Percutaenous jejunostomy

Technique very similar to the above with jejunostomy tube placement.

TIPS:

- Jejunum can be punctured under fluoroscopic guidance, however the bowel is mobile and may be difficult to puncture. This is much easier under CT guidance.
- Identify anterior loop near abdominal wall.
- Instill local anesthetic. Buscopan may be useful to reduce peristalsis.
- Puncture the jejunum and instill a small amount of air to confirm luminal position.
- Place T fasteners and use same needle to insert guidewire as above and dilate to appropriate size and exchange for feeding tube.
- Connect adapter and anchor to abdominal wall.

Further reading

Davies R.P, Kew J., West G.P. (2001) Percutaneous jejunostomy using CT fluoroscopy. A.J.R. **176**: 808–10.

Evans AL and Uberoi R, CT-Guided Jejunostomy Tube Insertion *AJR* 2005; **185**: 1369

Colonic stenting

The evidence base for this is weak.

Indications

Malignancy
- Acute obstruction as prelude to delayed surgery.
- Prophylactive if tight stricture on enema.
- Palliation in inoperable cancer (high risk/metastases).
- Fistula (consider removable stents) only with stricture.

Benign
- Should be avoided as stents will certainly migrate. But have been used to treat benign stricture temporarily where repeated balloon dilatation fails.

Contraindications
- Perforation.
- Uncooperative patient.
- Right colon lesions.

Preparation
- Bowel prep/rectal suppository/washouts rarely necessary.
- IV access.
- Single dose of broad spectrum antibiotic, i.e ciprofloxacin + metronidazole.

Equipment
- Colonoscope/stack with large channel for stent. Colonoscopic assistance speeds up the procedure. Length depends on site of lesion, the shorter the better.
- 10F Arrowflex sheath.
- Curved catheter, i.e. 5F Cobra, BMC, 5F headhunter.
- Bentson wire, standard and stiff treumo wire and long 260 cm Amplatz superstiff. Occasionally long ERCP type wires, i.e 400 cm JAG wire.
- Colonic stent are large bare stents >20 mm with different designs to prevent migration. Some are flared, i.e. Wallflex (Boston) or may be double barrelled stents, i.e. Nitis (Pyramed) or have irregular jagged surface, i.e. Memotherm (Bard), etc.
- Lubricant gel.

Imaging
- Idealy all patients should have colonsopic and contrast enema confirmation of tumour site/length and tightness of stricture or obstruction.
- CT is acceptable in planning cases.

Technique
Usually in the fluoroscopy room or mobile C arm.

Without colonoscope
- Patient left lateral semi-prone on fluoroscopy table.
- Lubricate BMC catheter combined with Bentson wire, negotiate fold in rectum into sigmoid.

- Air or standard diluted iodinated contrast can be used to distend and show lumen/stricture.
- Standard terumo wire/stiff wires are useful for direction control round bends and avoiding diverticula. Cobra catheter may have better shape in the rectosigmoid tumours and head hunter better for more proximal lesions, i.e descending colon.
- Standard terumo better for tortuous segments and stiff terumo often better for pushing through strictures.
- Oblique C arm to show stricture/occlusion tangentially and probe with terumo wire while rotating BMC catheter until stricture is crossed.
- Place catheter 5–6 cm beyond stricture, confirm position, exchange for stiff guidewire.
- Place arrow flex sheath, opacify length of stricture to assess stent size/length.
- Place stent of appropriate length with slightly more stent above the stricture than below to reduce migration risk. Ideally, there should be 3–4 cm of stent above the stricture and 2–3 cm below (Figure 14.9).
- Opacify stent length for peforation and opening.
- Do not routinely balloon dilate pre-or post stent to reduce risk of perforation. Rarely may need dilatation to insert stent. Use small balloon to allow stent delivery passage, i.e 10 mm.

With colosnoscopy

- The scope is negotiated to stricture. Not usually possible to pass across (if you can, usually don't need stent).
- Opacify the distal end of the stricture.
- Pass long guidewire up to 400 cm through the stricture. The 400 cm length is used if the working channel of the scope will not allow stent delivery passage (10F) and the scope needs to be exchanged for a long sheath.
- Opacify the proximal end of the stricture.
- Pass stent delivery through scope across lesion and deploy under fluoroscopy.
- If working channel unsuitable for direct stent, exchange scope for Arrowflex sheath over long wire and complete procedure as above (Figure 14.10).

Post procedure

- Monitoring of pulse, BP, respiration and assessment for possible perforation hourly for 4 hours and then 6 hourly for 24 hours.
- AP plain film at 12–24 hours to assess stent opening/migration/perforation.
- Stool softeners are advisable.

TIPS:
- Don't over distend the bowel as this makes finding the lumen more difficult. Sometimes aspiration or air/contrast aids in directing the guidewire.
- If difficult to get stiff wire to go up. Use small balloon above stricture to anchor position, i.e 5–6 mm.
- If catheter will not follow wire try using a 4F glide Cobra.
- If a lesion cannot be crossed while using a scope. Insert a long 6F MPA catheter (125 cm) through the scope to give direction and stiff terumo wire. Use plenty of saline to lubricate.
- If lesion still not crossed, try exchanging for a sheath and try with a 5F headhunter.

Technical success:	>94%
Clinical success	>91%
Complications:	23%
• Predominantly:	
• Perforation	<4%
• Migration	<12%
• Re-obsbruction	<8%

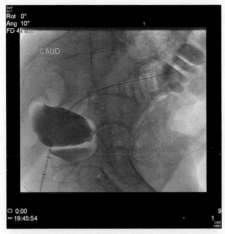

Figure 14.9 Colonic stent insertion using catheter and guidewire technique.

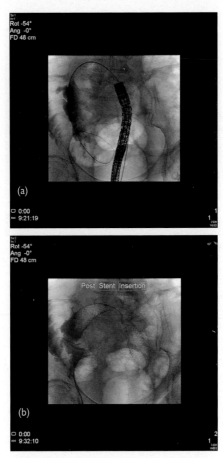

Figure 14.10 Colonic stent insertion with colonoscopic assistance.

Venous intervention

Endovascular treatment of DVT

Etiology: Venous thromboembolic disease is a common condition with a 1 year mortality rate of up to 25%. The etiologies of DVT fall into the general grouping of the Virchow's triad: endothelial injury, blood flow abnormalities, and hypercoagulability.

Treatment aims: To diminish the severity and duration of symptoms, prevent PE, minimize the risk of recurrent of venous thrombosis, and to prevent the post-thrombotic syndrome.

Conventional treatment: Anticoagulation with heparin followed by warfarin remains the conventional treatment. The majority of patients continue to experience some degree of venous obstruction indefinitely. The thrombus is removed incompletely in well over 50%

Thrombolytic therapy

Advantages

- Localized or systemic thrombolytic form of therapy available for treating DVT.
- Thrombolytic therapy has a high venous patency rate with a decreased incidence of chronic venous inefficiency and post thrombotic syndrome as well as better functioning and quality of life.

Potential complications

- High risk of haemorrhage.
- Unpredictability of the thromboablative effect and high possibility of patient exclusion due to stringent section criteria (see below).

Catheter directed loco-regional thrombolysis may reduce some of these complications and is superior in delivering high doses of thrombolytic agents directly into the venous thrombus.

Indications

- Patients with phlegmasia cerulean dolens.
- Venous gangrene.
- High risk of fatal PE.
- Extensive thrombus burden especially in the IVC or involving the ileo-femoral veins.
- Patients with propagation of thrombosis despite conventional therapy (see Figure 15.6).

Contraindication

Factors that increase the risk of bleeding including recent surgery, stroke, presence of aneurysms, and varices

Techniques

- Catheterization of the deep vein proximal to the thrombosis is performed using a 5F micropuncture set under US guidance using a 21G needle and a 0.018 guidewire. Perform a baseline ascending venography.
- A 5F hydrophilic end-hole catheter (Glidecath) over hydrophilic guidewire is then used to place the wire into the IVC through the thrombus.

- The Glidecath is then exchanged for a 90 cm catheter with a 50 cm infusion length (Unifuse).
- This catheter is then embedded into the thrombus prior to the initiation of thrombolytic therapy.

Infusion protocols: Numerous catheter protocols including 'bolus and wait', 'daily single dosing', and 'continuous infusion' techniques. The continuous infusion therapy overnight of TPA at 0.5–1 mg/hr remains the most popular option. The fibrinogen and PT values are obtained every 6 hours and maintained >100 mg/dl and <60 seconds. A low dose of heparin is also administered through a peripheral vein.

Assessment of outcome
- Venography after overnight thrombolytic infusion.
- Assess residual thrombus and look for venous stenosis or occlusion.
- In the absence of thrombus, the patients can be started on warfarin .
- Heparin infusion continued until the INR reaches therapeutic level.
- In the presence of extensive thrombus, the thrombolytic treatment is continued for a further 12 hours.

Percutaneous mechanical thromboectomy (PMT)
Indications
- For rapid clearance of thrombus.
- PMT where thrombus is resistant to catheter directed thrombolysis or conventional anticoagulation treatment.
- For patients with contraindications to continuous anticoagulation or prolonged thrombolytic therapy.
- Patients with critical venous thrombosis and rapid venous decompensation or in patients with thrombus involving the vena cava.

Complications
- Increased procedure time and radiation. Costly ($400–700/device).
- Potential endothelial damage and further propagation of DVT.

Categories
There are two main groups: rotational and hydrodynamic devices.
- **Rotational devices:** High speed rotating basket or impeller to break the thrombus into small particles which are naturally cleared trough the pulmonary circulation, i.e. Amplatz thrombectomy device, the Arrow –Terrotola device (Figure 15.1), Bacchus Fino device (Figure 15.2), and Cragg-Castaneda thrombolytic brush.
- **Hydrodynamic devices**: Retrogradely directed high speed saline is used to create a venturi effect with these devices. The high speed saline jet fragments the thrombus and the particles are then aspirated into the device. Due to the absence of rotatory blades, these devices cause less mechanical trauma to the thrombosed veins during thrombectomy.
- Examples include Oasis thrombectomy system, Angiojet, and Hydrolyzer.

Venoplasty and stenting

Indications
Venoplasty and venous stenting are important in anatomical vascular narrowing such as May Thurner syndrome, also in the management of haemodynamically significant residual thrombus after completion of thrombolysis, PMT or premature termination of thrombolysis due to intolerance or complication.

Complications
- Increased procedure time and radiation.
- Costly ($200–600/device). Venous rupture and haemorrhage.
- Require bigger venous access (6F or greater).

Technique
Refer to section on Renal Fistuloplasty.

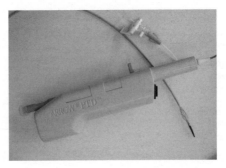

Figure 15.1 Arrow –Terrotola d rotational basket device used for venous mechanical thrombectomy.

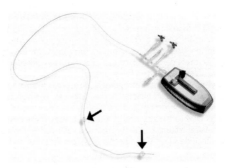

Figure 15.2 Trellis device from Bacchus which combines thrombolysis with mechanical maceration of clot between two occlusion balloons 20cm apart.

Vencava filters

Indications

Patents with DVT who have contraindication or resistant to conventional anticoagulation therapy.

Evidence of current literature

- In patients with a contraindication to anticoagulation.
- In patients who experience complications with anticoagulation treatment.
- In patients with recurrent VTE despite adequate anticoagulation.
- In patients with recurrent PE complicated by pulmonary hypertension.
- Pregnant pre delivery.
- Patients with free floating venous thrombus and in patients with DVT and limited cardiopulmonary reserve.
- Pre-operative high risk.

Contraindications

- Chronically thrombosed IVC or anatomical abnormalities preventing access to the IVC for filter placement are the two common contraindications to the placement of IVC filters.
- IVC <15 mm or >32 mm (may vary with device. Bird's nest filter for mega-cavas, i.e >32.

Complications

Occur in 4–11% of cases and include IVC thrombosis, increased recurrence of DVT, postphlebitic syndrome, filter migration, fracture and caval penetration, and guidewire entrapment.

Categories of filters

In the past IVC filters were divided into permanent and temporary devices. Currently almost all the new filters have the 'optional retrievable' facility. Examples of filters include Titanium Greenfield (Boston Scientific), Bird's nest (Guidant Corp), ALN (Figure 15.3) (Pyramed), Gunther tulip filter (Figure 15.4), Celect (Cook), TrapEase filter (Bard), and LGM/Vena Tech filter (B Braun).

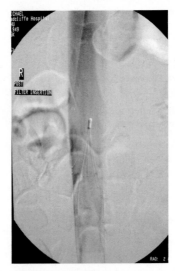

Figure 15.3 ALN IVC filter from Pyramed.

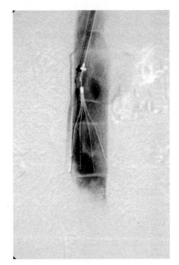

Figure 15.4 Tulip IVC filter from Cook.

Techniques

- Either via the femoral or internal jugular approach under flouroscopic and US guidance.
- Filters with low profile systems can also be placed through the anticubital vein approach.
- Access as previously described using the seldinger technique.
- Usually Right IJ or Right CF, some devices can be introduced from either Jugular/Femoral /Subclavian or Basilic venous access (i.e. Simon Nitinol).
- Placement of IVC filters using intravascular ultrasound or trans-abdominal ultrasound is also possible. May be a desirable option in ICU patient or patients with renal failure or contrast allergy.
- The standard placement of an IVC filter is, just below the renal veins, to avoid renal vein thrombosis in the event of filter occlusion.
- Catheter directed central venography is performed prior to filter placement to identify the origin of renal veins and to measure the caval diameter.

TIPS:
Alternatively, a curved catheter, i.e. Cobra can be used to enter and identify the renal veins and avoiding the need for contrast.

- Most filters have an upper and lower limit of IVC they can be used in. Bird's nest can be used in IVCs of up to 45 mm, others usually 30 mm.
- Suprarenal placement of filters may be considered in instances such as extension to the level of renal veins, ovarian vein thrombosis, or current pregnancy where filter placement below the renal veins is impossible or inadvisable .
- Techniques of deployment and removal vary between manufacturers.
- Usually requires introduction of a long sheath to just below the renal veins. Filter placed into the sheath and then pushed to the required level in the sheath.
- Filter then exposed by withdrawal of outer sheath. The Tulip and Celect filter legs or hook are attached and need separate release by depressing a thumb release button. These can be recovered and retrieved and moved before final release.

Suprarenal placement of filters
- Limited data on efficacy and safety of suprarenal filter placement. But have similar profiles to the infra-renal filters.
- Caution required as IVC thrombosis or filter occlusion will block renal vessels.
- Filters in the SVC can be considered in patients with upper extremity thrombus.

Removal of filters
- The removal of temporary IVC filters differs according to the brand of the filter inserted.
- Cooks Tulip, and Celect use a co-axial sheath and snare to grab the top hook and advance a sheath over the top dome to collapse the legs (Figure 15.5). ALN is removed using an identical technique but with graspers instead .The Opta-ease also has a hook but is removed from the femoral route.
- Filters can be left in the vena cava for 1–12 months depending on the manufacturer.
- Perform a central a venography prior to filter removal to demonstrate any presence of residual venous thrombus.
- Removal of the filter in the presence of significant central venous clot can subject the patient to PE.
- In the presence of thrombus consider thrombolysis before removing the filter, leaving it in situ permanently or removing it at a later date after anti-coagulation.

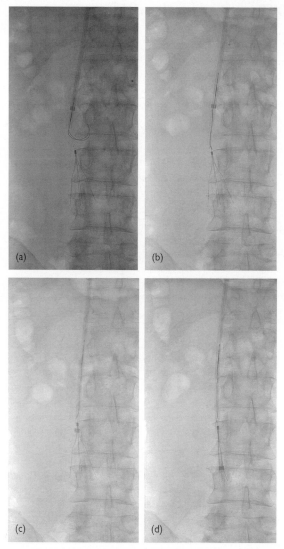

Figure 15.5 Shows the sequence of snaring the Tulip IVC filter (a,b) to advancing the inner then outer sheath over the body and legs to collapse the filter into the outer sheath. The filter is at no time pulled until the legs are well inside the sheath.

DVT treatment algorithm

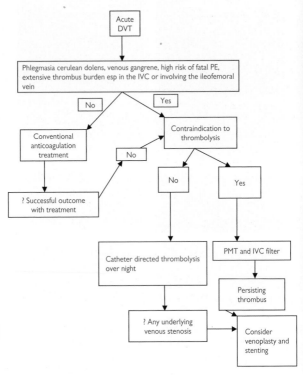

Figure 15.6 Diagramatic representation of using the lazer to occlude the long saphenous venous.

Endoluminal treatment of varicose veins

Background information

Varicose veins and its related symptoms constitute the most common vascular disorder of the lower limbs. It affects an average of 20% of people worldwide and the annual NHS treatment cost for varicose veins is estimated at £400–600 million.

Conventional treatment

Patients with symptomatic varicose veins are traditionally managed surgically under GA with ligation of the greater saphenous vein (GSV) at the saphenofemoral opening (SFO) +/– complete removal of GSV from the SFO.

Alternative treatment

Endovascular ablation of varicose veins by use of either radiofrequency (RF) or laser has been shown to have excellent long term success rate with lower recurrence than traditional surgical measures. The advantages of endovascular treatment include the avoidance of GA, earlier return to normal activities, minimal discomfort, shorter procedure time, and low recurrence rate.

Indications

Patients with symptomatic varicose veins include aching pain, leg heaviness, thrombophlebitis, external bleeding, ankle hyperpigmentation, venous ulcer, or cosmetic requests.

Complications

The complications of endoluminal treatment include altered leg sensation, cellulites, haematoma, and skin burn.

Technique

- The varicose veins are marked with the patient in the upright and recumbent positions.
- The area surrounding the GSV and distal tributaries are then infiltrated with a large volume of 0.1% diluted Lidocaine to produce 'tumescent anaesthesia'.
- The RF or laser catheter is then passed though the percutanoeus venous puncture site below the knee and the catheter tip is advanced to the GSO under ultrasound guidance.
- A near bloodless field is created especially in the case of RF ablation using the Esmark bandage.
- The radiofrequency generator is activated and the temperature is allowed to equilibrate at 85+- 3 degrees cel.
- The catheter is slowly pulled back at 2.5 cm/at 2–3 cm/second.
- In the case of laser ablation with a 5–600 Um laser the fibre is inserted into the vein within a protective sheath (Figures 15.7–15.8).
- Correct placement of laser fibre tip 2 cm distal to the SFJ is confirmed with US and viewing the He:NE aiming beam through the skin.
- The laser is activated in continuous firing mode with a slow mechanical withdrawal rate of 1 mm/s. Both hemoglobin absorbing wavelengths (810, 940, 980, 1064 nm) and collagen absorbing wavelengths (1320 nm) have been tried with the laser probes. The 1320 nm Nd; Yag laser

targeting the collagen in the vessel walls remains a popular choice as it seems to cause fewer side effects.

Choice of endovascular therapy

Both the laser and RF endoluminal techniques have similar success and complication rates. The laser systems are, however, becoming more popular compared to the RF method due to a number of practical advantages including greater efficiency in dealing with a large GSV system (20 mm), shorter procedure time, smaller access site (4F vs 6-dF for RF), and being cheaper.

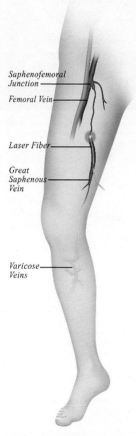

Saphenofemoral Junction

Femoral Vein

Laser Fiber

Great Saphenous Vein

Varicose Veins

Figure 15.7 'Schematic drawing showing slow-gradual withdrawal of laser from the saphenofemoral junction'. © Pyramed.

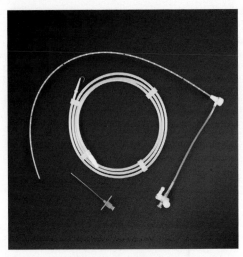

Figure 15.8 Basic equipment for access to perform lazer venous ablation. Access needle for an 0.35 J guidewire and long sheath. © Pyramed.

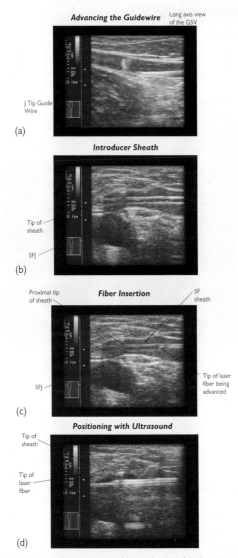

Figure 15.9 Ultrasound images showing (a) introduction of the J wire into the long saphenous vein, (b) followed by the sheath (c) and the laser is then advanced to just proximal to the SFJ and switched on. © Pyramed.

Treatment of SCVO

Aetiology

Benign

Thoracic aneurysm, goiter, vascular anomalies, benign tumor, granulomatous mediastinal disease, and the use of transvenous cardiac or indwelling venous access devices.

Malignant causes

(Malignant causes > benign, 10:1).

Mainly due to primary lung cancer (SCLC> NSCLC) (Figure 15.10). Less commonly lymphoma, metastatic disease, and other intrathoracic tumours such as mesothelioma and thymoma.

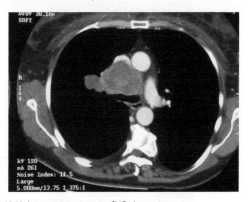

Figure 15.10 Lung carcinoma causing SVC obstruction.

Symptoms and signs of SVCO

These are neck swelling, distended veins over the chest, swelling of one or both arms, shortness of breath, hoarse voice, and headache. The symptoms are more severe when the SVC is obstructed below the entry of the azygos vein. The danger of SVCO (and risk of death) is increased by airway obstruction from laryngeal or bronchial oedema or coma from cerebral oedema.

Imaging of SVO

Imaging is vital in the assessment and treatment planning of SVCO. Non invasive investigations, i.e. CT or MRI examination are recommended as an initial assessment, although direct visualization of the venous obstruction by selective venography remains the gold standard.

Treatment of malignant SVO

Treatment is either purely symptomatic or directed at the underlying cause.

Conventional treatment

Traditional treatment for malignant SVCO includes systemic steroids, (prednisolone or dexamethasone), diuretics, and either radiotherapy (mostly for non-small cell cancers) or chemotherapy (mostly for small cell cancers). These therapies can take 2–4 weeks to show effectiveness with high complication rates. Surgical treatment is now rarely undertaken.

Endovascular treatment option

SVC stenting is now widespread in the management of occlusive venous disease. The placement of large expandable metal stents within the SVC allows for rapid restoration of the normal pattern of flow in the majority of patients.

Technique of SVC stenting

(see Figures 15.9–15.10)

- Usually carried out in a conscious patient under local anaesthesia.
- Venography is performed at the time of stenting to confirm the extent of the disease and define the landing zones for stenting.
- An access site from either basilic, jugular, subclavian or femoral veins can be used.
- The subclavian route may be a more advantageous.
- 5,000 units of heparin is given during the procedure.
- If there is extensive thrombus, thrombolysis or mechanical thrombectomy can be carried out to reduce the length of the obstruction and the risk of emboli.
- Using pre-shaped catheters (Cobra) and a variety of curved or hydrophilic guidewires, the stricture or obstruction is crossed from either above or below.
- A combined approach may sometimes be necessary to traverse tight lesions.
- Soft wires exchanged for 180 or 260 cm stiff guidewires.
- Pre dilatation of the stricture may be necessary, to allow the passage of the stent delivery system. It is vital that luminal re-entry is confirmed prior to balloon dilatation or stenting.
- Size the balloon to the vessel being dilated. Post dilatation of the stent may also be required to help fully expand stents if they fail to expand sufficiently in the subsequent 24–48 hours.

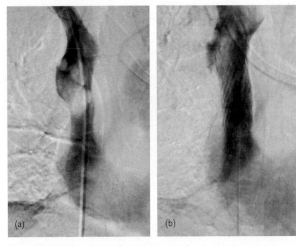

Figure 15.11 (a) Venogram confirm tight stricture due to extrinsic compression from the tumor. (b) Following successful stenting there is good venous flow into the right atrium.

Types of stents
A variety of stents have been used including balloon mounted and self expanding stents. The self expanding stents such as the Wallstent and the nitinol stents (Symphony, Boston Scientific, USA) are superior to the balloon mounted stents due to the ease of deployment and greater adaptability to the curves of the vessels. The Wallstent, however, does suffer from the disadvantage of unpredictable shortening during expansion which can continue for some days post procedure, resulting in uncovering of the obstructive lesion. Nitinol stents generally show minimal shortening during expansion.

Aftercare
Pulse, BP, Resp every 15 minutes for 1 hour then half hourly for 3 hours.
We do not routinely place our patients on long term anticoagulation unless it is for re-intervention and we manage patients with antiplatelets, i.e. clopidogrel and/or aspirin.

Complications
Complications include SVC rupture, haemorrhage, haemoptysis, epistaxis, pericardial tamponade, cardiac failure, recurrent laryngeal palsy, stent migration, pulmonary emboli, and groin haematoma.

Peripheral venous access and central venous catheters

Indications
- Patients who require parenteral nutrition.
- Long term antibiotic therapy, chemotherapy or haemodilaysis.
- Patients with difficult peripheral venous access.

Types of central lines
CVCs can be broadly categorized into four groups:
- Peripherally inserted central catheters (PICC).
- Temporary (non tunelled) CVCs,
- Long term (tunelled) CVCs.
- Implantable ports.

Regardless of access the optimal position for the tip of the line is at the junction or the right atrium to the SVC (usually two vertebral bodies below the Carina).

Peripherally inserted central venous catheters
Techniques
- Usually made of silastic or polyurethane materials and are usually 3–4F in size containing single or double lumens.
- Venous access with a PICC is achieved via the superficial veins of antecubital fossa, brachial, cephalic or basilic veins of the forearm.
- The basilic vein is frequently preferred due to an increased incidence of vaso-spasm of the cephalic vein and the close proximity of the brachial vein to the adjacent brachial artery.
- Lines are inserted using Seldinger technique using real time two dimensional ultrasound (2DUS).
- PICC systems specifically designed for radiologic placement such as the Vaxcel system (Boston Scientific) or RadPICC (Bard Access Systems) are commonly used for these purposes and are placed over a 0.018 wire.

Pros and cons of PICC lines
- PICCs are suitable for short (a few days) or long term (up to a year) use.
- Low risk of complications compared with other forms of CVCs.
- Veins identification is easier with peripheral access rather than the potentially more risky subclavian or jugular approaches.
- Peripheral access avoids the risk of pneumothroax and results in fewer infective complications.
- A significant disadvantage of PICC is more frequent occlusion due to their smaller diameter.
- The use of arm veins are for central venous catheterization is discouraged by the Dialysis Outcome Quality Initiative (DOQI) in patients with either current or pending haemodialysis in order to preserve veins for future haemodialysis access sites.

Temporary (non tunnelled) catheters

- Used for medication delivery.
- Central venous pressure monitoring.
- Short term haemodialysis.

They are different from long term catheters by having their exit ports in close proximity to the venous puncture site. Subclavian, jugular, and femoral venous routes can be used for these purposes.

Pros and cons

- Less time to insert.
- Cheap ($55).
- Increased risk of infection.
- Short term use only (<6 weeks).

Long term (tunnelled) central venous access

Tunnelled catheters can remain in place for many years and are often used for long-term total parenteral nutrition, chemotherapy or long term anti-biotic treatment. Examples of tunelled central venous devices include Hickman, Broviac, Groshong and Leonard catheters. Most of these include the polyester cuff as part of their design which has an anchorage and a microbial barrier function.

Pros and cons

- Lowers risk of infection.
- Can be used for long term purposes (>6 weeks).
- Long procedure time to insert.
- Cost (tunelled lines $190 vs Non tunnelled $55).

Ports

Implantable ports consist of a single or double lumen reservoir hub attached to a catheter. The intravascular part of ports is made of materials similar to other central venous catheters such as silicone or polyurethane. The thick injection membrane of the system made of siliastic material is secured in titanium or a plastic reservoir hub.

Techniques

- The catheter part of the port is inserted into a central vein in a similar manner to a tunnelled line using the Seldinger technique.
- The reservoir hub is then implanted surgically in the subcutaneous tissue, usually in the anterior chest wall at a site that is not apparent externally and is accessed using a non coring needle.

Pros and cons

- Used for long term access purposes.
- Lowest infection risk of all categories of central lines.
- Better cosmetic appearance as the injection hub is placed subcutaneously.
- Plastic ports produce minimal radiographic, MRI, and CT artifacts.
- However, they are more difficult to implant and are more costly.
- In addition they carry an additional risk of hidden extravasation of injected substances from needle dislodgement or incomplete needle placement

Venous access routes and techniques

Subclavian approach

- The subclavian vein lies behind the clavicle and immediately above the apex of the lung.
- Traditionally a 'blind' percutaneous approach was used to puncture the vessel.
- The subclavian vein can be punctured either by the supra or infraclavicular approach.
- With the infraclavicular method the skin should be punctured approximately 2 cm below and slightly lateral to the junction between the distal and middle thirds of the clavicle and the needle is directed towards the suprasternal notch in an approximately trajectory to the clavicle.
- The important landmarks for the supraclavicular approach are the clavicular insertion of the sternocleidomastoid muscle and the sternoclavicular joint.
- The site of the skin is punctured in the claviculosternomastoid angle, just above the clavicle and lateral to the insertion of the clavicular head of the sternocleidomastoid muscle.
- The supraclavicular approach is more meticulous with potentially higher complication risks and therefore should only be used by experienced operators.
- Subclavian catherization using the supra or infra clavicular approach is successful in 90–96% of cases.
- In addition to the anatomical landmark method described above, 2DUS guidance significantly decreases the risk of catheter placement failure and multiple attempts by up to 86%.

Internal jugular vein

Most commonly used site for gaining central venous access in an emergency situation, due mainly to its high success rate and lower complication rate as compared to its subclavian counterpart.

- The internal jugular vein can be punctured using either an anterior, central or a posterior approach.
- An important landmark in the anterior approach is the midpoint of the sternal head of the sternocleidomastoid muscle, approximately 5 cm from both the angle of the mandible and the sternum.
- The carotid artery is palpated and the needle is introduced 0.5–1 cm laterally. With the central approach the skin is punctured at the apex of the triangle formed by the two muscle bellies of the sternocleidomastoid muscle and the clavicle.
- The posterior approach uses the external jugular vein as a surface landmark. The needle is introduced 1 cm dorsally to the point where the external jugular vein crosses the posterior border of the sternoclidomastoid muscle.
- Internal jugular vein catherization has a success rate of 95–99% with few major complications.
- 2DUS guidance for cannulating the internal jugular vein is quicker and safer. Two dimensional ultrasound guidance can reduce failure of catheter placement and complication rates related to insertion by 86% and 57% respectively.

Femoral Vein

- Easiest of all central venous access punctures to perform but has a high incidence of complications, especially infection and thrombois, and therefore remains a less widely used route.
- The patient is placed in the supine position with the leg extended and slightly abducted at the hip.
- Femoral artery pulsation should be felt and the needle is inserted 1–1.5 cm medial to the artery and inferior to the inguinal ligament.
- The tip of the catheter is usually positioned just above the iliac bifurcation within the inferior vena cava.
- The risk of failed femoral catheter placement can be reduced by up to 71% using 2DUS.

Unconventional venous access routes

Percutaneous insertion into the IVC via a translumbar route or the external jugular vein, hepatic veins, and even intercostal veins can be performed if conventional routes are not accessible. Patients who most commonly require this type of access are those with prolonged central vein catherization for long-term haemodialysis or total parenteral nutrition.

Complications of the central venous access

Complications with the insertion of CVCs can be divided into those which occur at the time of catheterization (immediate) and those that develop at later stage (delayed).

Immediate complications

Pneumothorax

- 0-6%–12% and accounts for 25–30%.
- The internal jugular approach is associated with lower risk compared with subclavian central venous catheterization.
- PICC and femoral line insertions are not associated with increased pnumothorax risk.
- Symptomatic or large pneumothoraces may be treated with aspiration or chest drain insertion.

Inadvertent great vessel puncture/perforation

- Rupture of great vessels or cardiac perforation usually results in haemothorax, mediastinal haematoma, cardiac tamponade, or a combination of these. Can be fatal if unrecognized.
- Arterial punctures are more common with the jugular and femoral than with the subclavian approach.
- Bleeding from a punctured internal carotid or femoral arteries can usually be controlled by manual compression.
- Less frequently inadvertent carotid artery puncture can result in serious complications including airway obstruction, aortic dissection, arteriovenous fistula or cerebrovascular events.
- Bleeding from the subclavian vein can be occult and also can be difficult to control by manual pressure alone. Consequently the subclavian approach is less encouraged in patients with a bleeding tendency.
- Traditionally, uncontrollable arterial bleeding was managed surgically. However, increasingly interventional techniques have treatment of these sites with closure devices, balloon tamponade, and/or stent graft insertion in order to achieve adequate haemoastasiss.

Air embolism

This rare, lethal but preventable complication is often underestimated by practitioners. It occurs most commonly during the insertion of tunnelled catheters or ports immediately before intravascular catheter deployment. Air enters the vascular system between dilator removal and catheter insertion. Various manoeuvres can be performed to minimize this risk such as cramping the sleeve before catheter insertion or asking the patient to hum. Tiny air emboli probably occur quite commonly. When symptomatic the patient should be placed in the left lateral decubitus position and given 100% oxygen.

Catheter malposition

- Except with femoral central venous access, the tip of all other central venous access devices should lie outside the heart, just above the right atrium.
- Optimal positioning may not be achieved during insertion in the absence of image guidance in up to 25–40% of cases. With the use of 2DUS and fluroscopic guidance, accurate positioning of the tip can be achieved in 95–100% of cases.
- Positioning of the catheter tip in the cardiac silhouette is associated with an increased risk of cardiac tamponade and thrombosis.
- There is an increased incidence of thrombosis if the tip of the CVC remains in the proximal third of the SVC.
- Intracardaic tip position is associated with cardiac tamponade, dysrhythmias and infection.
- Malposition significantly less common with the jugular approach compared to the subclavain.
- Several methods of repositioning can be performed including forceful injection of saline or contrast into the CVC, direct manipulation by passing a guidewire through the catheter, and transfemoral manipulation using angiographic catheters and/or a loop snare.

Late complications

Infection

- Main complication following CVC insertion and occurs in up to 33% of the cases with an estimated mortality of 14–25%.
- Most infections have been found to arise from the migration of skin.
- Infection can occur with any type of intrvascular catheter and can manifest at the catheter exit site, in the tunnel or intravascularly.
- Exit site infections present with localized inflammation at the site of catheter exit through the skin. Most are due to *Staphylococcus epidermidis*. Frequently, these can be managed with local wound care and antibiotic treatment without the removal of the central venous access device.
- Tunnel or pocket infection is suppuration or induration related to the subcutaneous tunnel and often requires removal of the catheter to control the infection.
- Blood stream infection occurs most commonly in critically ill patients with no obvious localizing signs at the catheter site and no apparent focus of infection.
- Bacteraemia occurs more commonly with non tunelled catheters.

- CVCs appear less prone to cause infection if they are inserted via peripheral or subclavian veins rather than the femoral or internal jugular vein.

Venous stenosis

- Result of damage to the initma of the vein at the time of CVC insertion.
- The left sided internal jugular vein approach results in fewer stenoses than the right.
- The subclavian veins have the highest incidence of stenosis.
- Ultrasound, venography, linograms, CT, and MIR imaging can all be useful in the diagnosis of venous stenosis.

Fibrin sheath and thrombus formation

- Most common cause of catheter dysfunction, occurs in 5–10% of patients.
- Thrombus and fibrin sheaths can function as one way valves allowing catheter flushing but not aspiration.
- Thrombosis is more likely to occur when a small lumen vein is chosen for CVC insertion. This could explain why thrombosis is more frequent with PICCs compared to other forms of CVCs.
- The subclavain venous catheterization may carry the lowest risk of catheter related thrombus.
- Infusion of tissue plasminogen activator into the catheter is the first line treatment for dysfunction due to fibrin sheath (lock in 5–10 mg rTPA for 10 min repeat x3).
- If this fails catheter exchange over a guidewire, by balloon angioplasty or by stripping the fibrin sheath off the catheter using a loop snare.
- Effective flushing and prophlactic use of warfarin or heparin can reduce the risk of catheter related thrombosis.

Further reading

Ganeshan, A., Warakaulle, D.R., Uberoi, R. (2007) Central venous access. *Cardiovasc Intervent Radiol.* **30**(1): 26–33. Review.

Janssen, M.C.H., Wollersheim, H., Janssen, Schultze-Kool, L.J., Thien T.H. (2005), Local and sytemic thrombolytic therapy for acute deep vein thrombosis. *Netherland J of Medicine* **3**: 81–90.

Uberoi, R. (2006) Quality assurance guidelines for superior vena cava stenting in malignant disease. *Cardiovasc Intervent Radiol.* **29**(3): 319-22.

Interventional radiology in management of gynecological disease

Uterine leiomyomas (fibroids)

This is the most common benign tumour of the female genital tract. It affects 25% of women of reproductive age. It has a higher incidence in the African-Caribbean population. Most are asymptomatic. Counselling with a gynaecologist should be carried out.

Indications
Sympptomatic patients with fibroids:
- Uterine bleeding.
- Pelvic pain.
- Urinary or bowel obstructive symptoms.
- Infertility and miscarriage (other causes must be excluded first, also consider myomectomy).

Contra-indications
- Current or recent genital tract infection.
- Where patient would not consider hysterectomy under any circumstances (complication of procedure).
- Serious doubt of diagnosis.

Relative contra-indications
- Narrow stalked pedunculated subserous fibroids.
- Procedure should be performed in the early or follicular phase of the cycle (first 10 days) if patient unsure of adequate contraception.
- Pre- planning with MR and MRA is extremely valuable and is a baseline for follow up. Will demonstrate large ovarian arterial supply.
- UAE is performed under conscious sedation with monitoring/oxygen.
- IV access and planned analgesic regime, i.e. PCA with non steroidal anti-inflammatory drugs.
- Single dose of antibiotics with combination of metronidazole with cephalosporin, a quinolone (ciprofloxacin) may be helpful (limited data).
- Femoral approach (see 📖 Chapter 5) and 5F sheath placed. Some adovacate bilateral approach for speed.
- An aortogram is useful for as assessing anatomy (Figure 16.1).
- Use frequent angiograms/roadmap facilities to guide procedure.
- A curved catheter (i.e. 4F glide Cobra) is selectively introduced in combination with a curved terumo wire, into the uterine artery to occlude the blood supply (Figure 16.2). Micro catheters/microwires may be required for difficult cases.

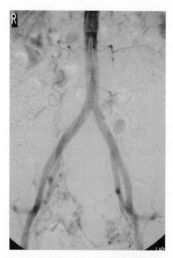

Figure 16.1 Aortogram with a 5F pigtail catheter, from the right femoral artery access showing large right ovarian artery and uterine arteries.

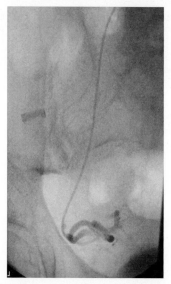

Figure 16.2 4F gluide cobra catheter from contra-lateral approach into the right uterine artery.

- Various embolic agents (350–750 microns) including polyvinyl alcohol (PVA), gelfoam, and trisacryl microspheres are currently available. Embospheres are more superior to spherical PVA.
- Intermittent injections to confirm stagnation of contrast flow and ensure no reflux should be performed.

TIPS:

Bilateral femoral approach quicker and lower radiation than single side approach.

Large ovarian arteries may also need embolization (Figure 16.3); usually delayed to assess outcome of uterine artery embolization first.

- Closure devices have been used but simple compression is adequate.

Technical success
96–98% with symptomatic improvement in 85–90%.

Complications
In 5–7%.

Immediate
- Haematoma.
- Dissection.
- Thrombosis.
- Dissection.
- Pseudoaneurysm.
- Embolization of non target organs.

Early (<30days)
Post embolization syndrome (usually first 2 weeks) pain, nausea, fever, flu like raised inflammatory marker, and WC count. If prolonged raise concern of infection.

Late (30 days)
- Vaginal discharge 16% at 12 months.
- Fibroid expulsion 10%.
- Amenorrhoea 1–2% , 7.3% in >45 years.
- Sexual function 12% at 12 months.
- Infection 0.5%.

Hysterectomy may be required in 2.9%.

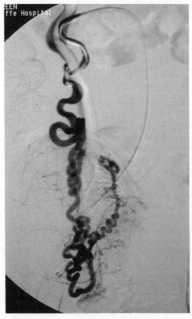

Figure 16.3 Selective right ovarian arteriogram using a 5F SOS Omni catheter, prior to embolization.

Pelvic congestion syndrome

Chronic pelvic pain (CPP) is defined as pain in the lower abdomen or pelvis with a duration of more than 6 months, not exclusively cyclical or intercourse related and not usually relieved by narcotic analgesics. CPP accounts for 10–40% of all gynaecological referrals and pelvic congestion syndrome (PCS) is one of its causes.

Aetiology

- Multifactorial: absence of ovarian vein valves, external vascular compression, including the nutcracker syndrome (left renal vein is compressed between the aorta and the superior mesenteric artery), secondary ovarian vessel congestion due to portal hypertension or acquired inferior vena cava syndrome.
- Indications: symptomatic patients often fail medical therapy with large veins and reflux (veins usually >8 mm, with dilated uterine veins and cross flow).
- The procedure is usually carried out at the time of diagnostic venography (Figure 16.4).
- Femoral or Jugular vein approach: jugular easier. Catheter tracking is easier with a jugular approach, however patients don't always like this.
- 5F sheath, standard wire then hydrophilic wire (Terumo), 4F SIMMS 2/Cobra catheter from the femoral and MPA from the Jugular. Right ovarian cannulated directly off IVC and the left off the renal vein.

TIPS:

Be aware of variants, i.e. both veins of IVC or right off the right renal vein. Tip the table with head up 30 degrees or more to help distend veins/valsalva and inject into the renal veins to assess reflux. Embolize in this postion to prevent reflux of sclerosant.

- Place catheter as distal as possible and inject sclerosant slowly followed by long coils, i.e. Nester's (Cook's, UK), etc. up to the origin of the veins. These can be forced out with a jet of saline in a 2 ml syringe or pushed with a Bentson wire. The latter allows more accurate coil placement. Don't fire out near the renal vein.

TIPS:

Connect two 2 ml syringes onto a three way tap. Cut up gel foam into tiny pieces and place in the syringe by removing the back plunger and replace. Put 2 mls of STD into the other syringe and then inject back and forward to form slurry for injection.

Rarely, a co-axial microcatheter may be needed to get very distally.

Technical success

In 98–100%, recurrence <8%. Improvement of symptoms occurs within the first two weeks and is recorded in 70–85% of patients.

Complications

In <4%, including ovarian vein thrombophlebitis, recurrence of varices, migration of embolic material, and radiational exposure to ovaries.

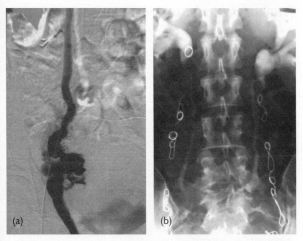

Figure 16.4 (a) Right Ovarian venogram using a 5F SIMMS 2 catheter from a right femoral vein access. (b) Following successful bilateral ovarian vein embolization using coils and gelforam /sclerosant mix.

Post partum haemorrhage

This is a major cause of maternal morbidity and mortality in 2–11% of delivery. Defined as excessive blood loss (>500 mls) in a vaginal delivery and at least 1000 mL following caesarean section or a 10% reduction in haematocrit between admission and the post partum period of up to six weeks. Uterine atony is the commonest cause. Others include lower genital tract laceration, placenta acreta, retained placental products, rupture or inversion of the uterus, and coagulopathy.

When medical measures are unsuccessful, surgical alternatives include:
• Bilateral ligature of the hypogastric.
• Uterine arteries.
• B-Lynch sutures.
• Intra-uterine balloon dilatation.
• In refractory cases hysterectomy.

UAE is an alternative. The procedure is as above for UAE. Non-selective anterior division or internal iliac embolization is also acceptable.

It may also be used to treat ante partum hemorrhage and for prophylactic purposes (e.g. prior to delivery when the fetus is dead or has an ectopic position or displays disease incompatible with life during the second and third trimesters of pregnancy).

Technical success
In >90%.

Complications
In <9%, similar to fibroid embolization and includes fever, vascular perforation, transient buttock ischemia, pelvic abscess, groin haematoma, and bladder gangrene.

Uterine arterio-venous malformation (AVM)

AVMs of the uterus are rare and can be congenital or acquired. Gestational trophoblastic disease remains the commonest cause of acquired uterine AVM. Others include trauma, previous uterine surgery, endometrial carcinoma, removal of intrauterine contraceptive devices, and exposure to diethylstilbestrol.

It presents with episodes of severe vaginal bleeding, infertility, and/or anemia which fail to respond to medical and hormonal therapy. The diagnosis is often made either using MRI, hystroscopy or selective arteriography.

It was historically managed by hysterectomy with or without internal iliac artery ligation. Transcatheter embolization of uterine AVMs is an alternative conservative option. It was first described by Forssman et al. in 1982 and is now considered the treatment of choice.

- Technique as for UAE.
- Branches from the predominant uterine artery supplying the AVM are embolized first.
- Selective angiography of the contralatral uterine artery is subsequently performed and embolization is performed in the presence of any persistent vascular supply to the malformation.

Success
In >95%.

Complications
In <4%, i.e. transient paresthesia with paralysis of the left arm and persistent blue coloration of the cervical os and vagina.

Fallopian tube recanalization

Infertility affects 8–20% of couples. Fallopian tube obstruction is a recognized cause. The absence of bilateral peritoneal passage of contrast at hysterosalpinography (HSG) is either due to tubal spasm or occlusive tubal disease (i.e. infection, endometriosis, surgery, salpingitis isthimica nodosa, etc). Tubal spasm generally relaxes after a few minutes without any further intervention.

In the presence of proximal or mid tubal obstruction, selective salpingography and tubal recanalization can be attempted by interventional radiologists.

- Usually performed under conscious sedation on an out patient basis.
- IV access and single dose of antibiotic may be given.
- Monitoring and oxygen during sedation.
- A pre-curved 5 or 4F catheter is passed though the normal HSG catheter and manipulated into the tubal ostium.

TIPS:

Alternatively, a long 10F sheath (Arrow flex) can be used with a speculum.

- A 0.35 hydrophilic guide wire is advanced (Terumo) through the 5–4F catheter and using torque movement and a slight exertion of pressure the occluded point is negotiated to restore normal peritoneal spillage.
- If a proximal tubal stenosis persists or recurs, a balloon tuboplasty may be considered.

Success

Selective salpingography is possible in more than 90% of cases and establishing tubal patency occurs in 50% of patients.

Complications

In 0–13% including 5% perforation, also small tubal tears without any major clinical sequeale, and minor bleeding up to 48 hours.

20–25% of infertile couples conceive successfully within six months. Ectopic pregnancy occurs in 4.5–15%.

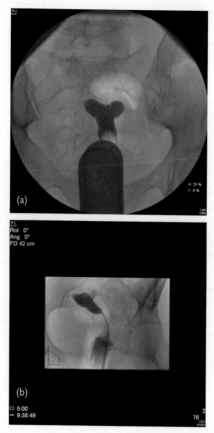

Figure 16.5 (a) Hyterosalpingogram showing bilateral fallopian tube occlusions (b) with successful recanalization using a 4F Cobra catheter and Terumo guidewire.

Recanalization of the cervical os

Occlusion of the cervix can be either congenital or acquired. Congenital forms of cervical occlusion have obstructive components with an abnormal cervix, congenital webs or tissue blocks. The cervical os may also be stenosed or occluded from a malignant process or due to previous surgery, cervical conization, radiotherapy or infection.

Re-establishing patency of the cervical os can be achieved by puncturing the central area of the cervix using a trocar containing needle under ultrasound guidance. A guidewire is then passed through the needle into the uterine cavity. Selective dilators and nitinol self expandable stents can then be used to recreate the cervical os.

Drainage of pelvic abscesses and collections

Pelvic collections and abscesses can be drained percutaneously through anterior abdominal transrectal or transvaginal approaches under image guidance using Seldinger or trocar techniques. The transabdominal route may be difficult due to a long distance to the pelvic lesion, or intervening intestine, bladder and/or reproductive organs. The posterior transgluteal approach is shorter but tends to be more painful and exposes the patient to an increased risk of neurovascular injury.

The trasvaginal or transrectal routes are ideally suited to pelvic abscess drainage due to the proximity of the vagina and rectum to many of pelvic fluid collections. The main consideration with the transrectal or transvaginal route is the potential to cause super-infection of sterile fluid collections due to the non sterile route of access. Therefore, care must be taken to assess the fluid collection adequately using CT or MRI imaging before drainage.

Technique

Preparation
- Consent, clotting, and IV access.
- Monitoring and oxygen.
- Conscious sedation, local anaesthetic (lidocaine 1%) and antibiotic cover.

Equipment
- TV probe (ideally with a guide, a peel-away sheath attached to the probe can be used but is more cumbersome).
- Large speculum (large condom).
- Long needle 20 cm+length >18 gauge (Chiba).
- Stiff guidewire (Amplatz stiff).
- Dilaters 6F+, 8–16F locking pigtail drain.

Procedure:
- Lithotomy position with two pillows under the buttocks to raise introitus.
- Insert speculum and localize collection/target with US with attached needle guide.

- Insert needle (Figure 16.6a), instill 5–10 mls lidocaine,puncture target, insert guidewire, exchange for dilator and then drain (Figure 16.6b).

TIPS:

Use the onestick drain (Boston Scientific) over the wire with the central trochar removed. The metal stiffener makes it much easier to place the drain at a distance. Very useful for all drains.

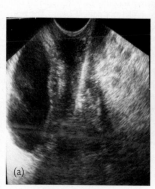 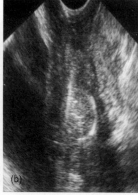

Figure 16.6 (a) Needle into a pelvic collection using transvaginal approach (b) with successful placement of 8F locking pigtail drain.

Image guided aspiration/biopsy of ovarian or adnexal lesions

Aspiration or biopsy of adnexal and ovarian lesions with malignant features are of low value and definitive surgical treatment must therefore be sought. There are a small subgroups of patients with adnexal or ovarian lesions who are ideal candidates, i.e. women with postoperative symptomatic seromas or lymphoceles, pregnant women with symptomatic ovarian cysts, and patients with previously confirmed ovarian malignancy with recurrent symptomatic cysts, or patients who are high risk surgical candidates. They can be aspirated or biopsied percutaneously or trans-vaginally using ultrasound under conscious sedation on an out patient basis. The trans-vaginal route has the disadvantage of being semi-sterile and should only be used for solid lesions or cystic lesions that can be completely aspirated to reduce the risk of infection. When biopsying predominantly cystic masses, care must be given to aspirate the fluid component completely prior to acquisition of the tissue sample in order to reduce the risk of infection.

The disadvantages of this technique include high recurrence rates, low diagnostic success rates, and an increased risk of tumor seeding.

Technique as for drainage except long biopsy aspiration or cutting needle used.

Embolization techniques

Imaging

Equipment

- High quality angiography equipment with DSA. Good road mapping or fluoro fade very helpful. Rotational angiography useful in complex vascular anatomy
- Duplex useful for puncture and lesion guidance.
- Preparatory vascular imaging with multidetector CT or contrast enhanced MR useful in planning embolization procedure.

Catheters

- 5–6F sheath. This allows a conventional 4–5F catheter and a microcatheter to be used. It is important to be able to remove each part of the system and maintain access.
- 4–5F catheter hydrophilic or conventional. End hole only.
- Microcatheter. Hydrophilic with guide wire that can be manually shaped most useful. Flow guided catheters occasionally useful in tortuous vessels.
- If the access is particularly tenuous or critical, e.g. visceral vessels or head and neck, a long guiding catheter in the vessel origin may be helpful. Curved tips or straight tips depending on anatomy.
- Direct puncture needles. Useful if trans-arterial access is not possible. Butterfly, angiography needle or spinal needle chosen depending on depth.
- Occlusion balloons or tourniquet may be useful in reducing flow through a lesion.

Embolic agents

Particles

(see Figure 17.1)

Such as PVA (Cook, UK)/Embospheres. Useful in embolization of solid tumours, e.g. fibroids, renal or hepatic tumours.

Pros
- Effective embolization of vascular bed.
- Temporary.
- Catheter does not have to be at lesion as particles flow antegradely.

Cons
- Not permanent.
- Not completely controllable as particles flow antegradely.
- As lesion fills up, flow slows down and more likely to reflux particles into non-target areas.

> **TIPS:**
>
> Use microcatheter to select only target area. Can be helpful to inject under DSA to detect reflux.

- Size. Smaller particles (100–300 μm) produce more effective embolization, but more necrosis (Figure 17.1). Larger particles (300–500) or (500–700) treat bigger area but produce less necrosis.
- Microspheres or beads have more uniform size than particles and may produce more complete necrosis. These agents are now available with drug coating and may be useful in tumour embolization.
- Gelfoam (temporary occluding agent). Comes as powder (40–60 μm) for distal embolization (uncommonly used) or as small sheets. The latter are cut longitudinally and then transversely to make little pledgets. These can be mixed with contrast to soften and make visible by placing in a gallipot of 20 mls of contrast and drawn up into a syringe (5 mL usually).
- TIP or take the plunger off the 5mL syringe, put in the dry pledgets and replace plunger. Connect to a 3 way tap with another 5 mL syringe of contrast and push in and out to make a slurry which can then be injected directly into the patient. This can also be used to embolize the tract following a liver biopsy or PTC.
- Or make into little bullets, push into the barrel of the catheter with the stiff end of the wire and fire out with a little saline using a 2ml syringe.

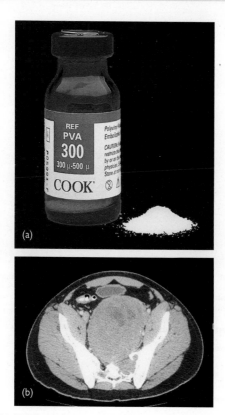

Figure 17.1 (a) PVA embolization particles. © Cook. (b) Large pelvic tumor.

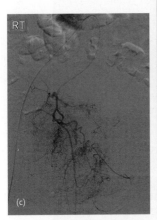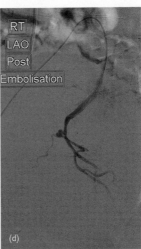

Figure 17.1 *(Continued)* (c) Pre embolization angiogram shows multiple small tumor vessels (d) Using small 300 micron particles the tumor has been embolized distally to produce maximum necrosis, but the proximal larger vessels remain patent.

Liquid embolic agents

Glue (Histoacryl)®

Pros
- Highly effective.
- Fast.
- Does not require normal clotting.
- Visible.

Cons
- Very fast and difficult to control.
- Needs special syringes but can use plastic syringes and tubes which need to be discarded immediately after injection.
- May not diffuse down all feeding vessels.
- Theoretical (but very small) risk of catheter sticking.

TIPS:

- Always use microcatheter as access can be maintained.
- Have an experienced assistant.
- Dilute 1:2 with lipiodol to delay polymerization (put lipiodol in a glass bottle until ready to be used as it corrodes the plastic).
- Use prepared products such as Glubran® (Radiologic Sheffield, UK) which are slower to polymerize.
- Use very small volumes (0.05–0.1 mls) per injection.
- Chase with dextrose 50%.
- Do not pull catheter sharply after injection. Risk of catheter sticking small and risk of non-target embolization high.

Alcohol

Pros

- Inexpensive.
- Effective in vascular malformations and also used for treating cysts.
- Permanent.

Cons

- Non-radio-opaque.
- Painful need to use sedation and analgesia and may require GA.
- Neurotoxic.
- Pulmonary hypertension.
- Causes cell death by dehydration and will cause severe tissue necrosis if extravasated.

TIPS:

- Alcohol is a useful agent in treating the nidus in arteriovenous malformations.
- Not viscous so diffuses well through nidus.
- Can be used via direct puncture into nidus.
- Assess the volume to inject by small alloquots of contrast until it leaks out into the circulation to assess volume required to be injected.
- Can be used with occlusion balloon or tourniquet to increase time in contact with nidus.

Onyx®

Alcohol copolymer/tantalum suspension.

Pros

- Very controllable.
- Radio-opaque.
- Permanent.

Cons

- Expensive.
- Slow to deploy.
- Long DSA times.
- Painful, requires GA.
- Needs special DMSO resistant catheters.

STD Sodium tetradecyl sulphate (STD Pharmaceuticals, Hereford, UK):
- Detergent sclerosant.
- Useful in sclerotherapy of low flow lesions.
- Used in venous outflow of high flow lesions.
- Can be mixed with air and lipiodol to form foam which fills large volume and promotes stasis.
- Absolute contraindication to arterial injection.

Devices

Coils (Figure 17.2).

Pros
- Permanent.
- Controllable.
- Huge range of sizes.
- Deploy by conventional or microcatheter.
- Often retrievable if deployed incorrectly.

Cons
- Can only deploy at catheter tip, won't flow away.
- May not travel well in tortuous catheters.
- Vessels often re-canalize unless well packed.
- Often require many coils to pack vessel.

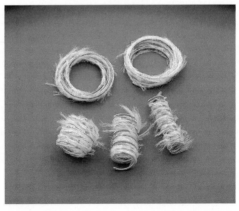

Figure 17.2 Coils with cotton fibres to increase thrombogenicity. © Cook.

TIPS:

- Safer to use via microcatheter.
- Use smaller and shorter coils than predicted.
- Most problems from large long coils which fail to deploy coiled up.
- Pack the vessel as full as possible, i.e. push them into a tight bundle.
- Do not stop until vessel occluded and flow stopped. Delayed occlusion will rarely occur and recanalization more likely.
- If positioning is critical consider detachable coils which can be deployed and removed if not perfect.

Methods for deploying coils

- Load coil well into the barrel of the catheter by putting the coil container barrel tight against the lumen (some coil containers have luer lock mechanism to keep in position) and use either the pusher supplied or still end of the Benston to introduce the coil 4–5 cm into the catheter, before formally deploying
- Use pusher for microcatheter or Bentson wire for 0.35 lumen catheters, give more precise deployment and allow coil packing.
- Firing with saline. Impressive and quick but more dangerous. Need very stable subelective position. Use 1 or 2ml syringes filled with saline and inject with moderate force. If you inject too hard, the catheter and sometimes the coil will recoil out of the vessel !

Amplatzer devices

(see Figure 17.3)

Will fit through 6 or 8F guiding catheters depending on size 8–20mm diameter.

- Very good in large AV fistula and for other large vessels.
- Controllable.
- Expensive (but cheaper than multiple coils for occluding large vessels, i.e. internal iliac prior to EVAR).

Deployment requires a 6–8F guiding catheter/sheath with a Tuhoy-Bohrst, shape dependant on the site of delivery. It comes attached to a stiff 0.35 wire with screw attachment to the tip. To prepare the device is extruded into a pot of heparinized saline to remove all the air and then retracted under water into the housing container.

When the guiding catheter is at the desired delivery point, the Amplatzer is introduced through the Tuhoy-Bohrst and pushed with the stiff attached deployment wire and extruded into the desired point. If unsatisfactory it can be pulled back in and repositioned or released by rotating the wire anticlockwise to release the device.

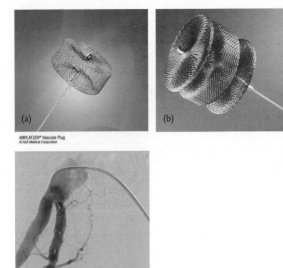

AMPLATZER® Vascular Plug
© AGA Medical Corporation

Figure 17.3 (a) Original Amplatzer and (b) the new Amplatzer device. The new device is more thrombogenic with more planes of occlusion. The devices need to be sized approximately 40% larger than the target vessel. When pushed out of the guiding catheter it will form a spindle shape but can be completely withdrawn or pulled back with the catheter. If in a good position it is released by unscrewing the thread which attaches the apex of the device give accurate deployment (c) as shown during II embolization pre EVAR. © Amplatzer Medical.

Specific indications

GI haemorrhage (see 📖 Chapter 4)
- Preliminary multidetector CT very useful in location of bleeding.
- Catheter C1 or S1.
- Guiding catheter in difficult anatomy.
- Transbrachial approach useful in vessels with profound caudal direction.
- Most upper GI bleeding comes from vessels with dual supply from celiac and SMA:
  • Need for superselective catheterization.
  • Aim to embolize both sides of bleeding point (front and back door) (Figure 17.4).
  • Microcoils most controllable embolic material.
  • Vital to pack vessel with coils (Figure 17.5), and observe absence of flow.
  • In catastrophic bleeding glue 0.05–0.1 mls can be life saving as bleeding will be halted immediately.
  • Intestinal ischaemia uncommon in stomach and duodenum/jejunum. More common in large bowel.

Vascular malformations
- Accurate diagnosis vital. Usually clear on history and examination.
- Duplex helpful in clinic situation.
- MRI best technique for extent of lesion.
- Categorize lesions into low and high flow.
- Invasive angiography only as part of treatment episode.
- Low flow lesions respond well to sclerotherapy with alcohol or STD.

TIPS:
- Preliminary angiogram – measure lesion volume.
- Assess venous drainage and control with tourniquet or occlusion balloon.
- Fill lesion with 1% or 3% STD foam until just into draining veins.
- Compression of lesion.
Repeat at 4–6 weekly intervals.

High flow lesions
- Probably best left to specialist referral centres.
- Accurate and complete angiography as first stage.
- Assessment of number of feeding and draining vessels.
- Arteriovenous – single inflow and outflow. Can be cured with obliteration of nidus.
- Arteriolovenous. Multiple feeders. Single outflow. Transvenous obliteration of nidus may be successful.
- Arteriolovenulous. Multiple feeders and outflow. Palliation and control only possible.

Agents
- Usually liquid agents, glue alcohol and onyx.
- STD must not be used on arterial side as it can foam and produce profound ischaemia.

- Full informed consent vital as complications will occur. Important to balance risks and benefits.
- No place for coiling of feeders as this will make subsequent access difficult or impossible.
- First procedure has best chance of success.
- Transvenous or percutaneous access to nidus useful. Production of stasis with tourniquets or occlusion balloon very useful.

Pulmonary AVM

- Only should be treated in specialist centres.
- Preliminary multidetector CT for anatomy.
- Rotational angiography useful.
- Operator should be familiar with use of Amplazter devices and detachable coils.

Treatment of femoral false aneurysm

Commonly after coronary angioplasty (large catheters and high doses of anti-coagulant)/poor compression /failure of closure device.

Treatment options

- **Nothing**: although many will self thrombose risky if the aneurysm enlarges and ruptures.
- **Compression using ultrasound guidance**: Works well if there is a narrow neck which can be compressed to stop flow into aneurysm. Can take 15–60 minutes and is painful both to patient and operator! May need analgesia. Re-scan in 24 hours.
- Alternatively, mark neck with Duplex and use a compression device, i.e. Femstop
- **Thrombin injection**. Now currently only TISSEEL® preparation available. Mix calcium chloride with the thrombin powder provided. Use 1 or 2 mls syringe. Puncture aneurysm under US control (do not aspirate) and inject 0.1 ml aliquots with color Doppler to confirm when thrombosis complete (Figure 17.6). **Do not over-inject as this will result in thrombin extravasation with femoral emboli/clot**. 2 mls adequate but maybe more if large. Re-scan in 24 hours. Recurrence reported rarely some weeks later. Anaphylaxis/emboli/occlusion/infection recognized complications.
- Surgery.

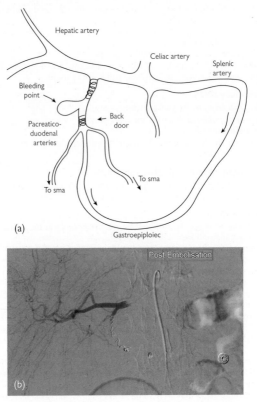

Figure 17.4 (a) Diagramatic representation of the celiac circulation. It is important when there are multiple collateral pathways that the back door to aneurysms or bleeding points is closed otherwise it will result in treatment failure.

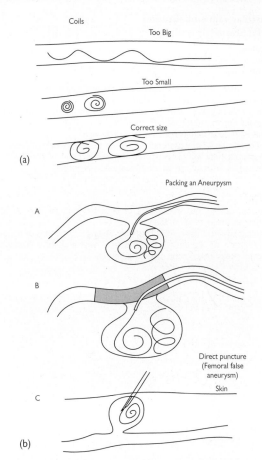

Figure 17.5 (a) When using coils it is important to size to the vessel so that they just begin to coil so that they can be compacted together to form a tight ball. If too large a coil is used it will not pack down and thrombose and similarly if they are too small they will migrate distally.

(b) When coiling an an aneursym directly detachable coils can be used (as for cranial aneurysms) and delivered directly into the aneurysm (A) or a cage can be made by stenting across the neck of the aneurysm and then placing coils through the struts (B) and sometimes direct puncture into the aneurysm can be performed with a needle and 0.35 or 0.14 micro-coils depending on the size of the needle (C).

Testicular vein embolization

(see 📖 Chapter 11)

Indications

- Pain/discomfort.
- Subfertility.

This is almost identical in technique to the treatment of pelvic venous congestion in woman (see 📖 Chapter 16).

- Key points remain to embolize as distally as possible right down to the inguinal ring to reduce risk of failure/recurrence (Figure 17.7). Layer coils right up to within 1–2 cm of the renal vein.
- There may be several branches or a single testicular vein with several tributaries these will all need to be occluded, separately if necessary.
- Although sclerosant can be used, most often only coils.

TIPS:

The vein can go into spasm very easily, avoid multiple catheter/wire exchanges and irritation of the vein.

If there is spasm it may resolve by simply waiting 4–5 minutes or try glyceryltrinitrate 100 µg directly into the vein, wait another 4–5 minutes, repeat if necessary or come back another day.

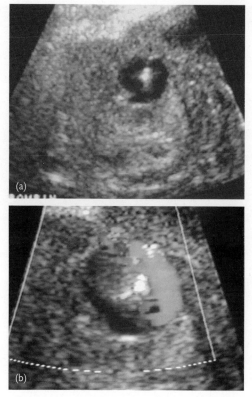

Figure 17.6 Needle into a femoral false aneurysm prior to thrombin injection (a) and (b) immediately after 0.2mls of thrombin showing clot formation around the needle.

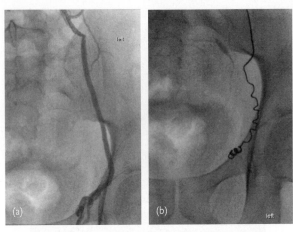

Figure 17.7 Embolization of testicular vein using platinum coils.

Trauma

(see 📖 Chapter 4)

- Can be life saving. Speed is important. Don't try to be too selective if it is taking a long time, i.e. complete internal iliac occlusion will often be fine, if there is one on the other side.
- Preliminary CT now investigation of choice, will often identify organ involved if not the actual bleeding point (Figure 17.8a) and guide angiography/embolization (Figure 17.8b–c).
- Beware of more than one vessel supplying the territory.
- Coils generally used although gel foam pledgets are also excellent materials for this. Glue useful in catastrophic haemorrhage.
- For bowel injury important to take acount of collaterals (so called back door which allow persistent bleeding). See also section on GI bleeding.
- Covered stentgrafts – useful on the shelf for large ruptures.

Complications

Beware of non target embolization. Coils can be retrieved but not always and not liquid or particulate agents. Patients should be warned of this!

- Be cautious, take your time and pay meticulous attention to technique. Use multiple views and contrast injections between embolizations to make sure where the agents are going.
- Tissue necrosis and abscess formation may occur if complete tissue infarction is obtained, particularly using liquids and particles. May need antibiotics.
- Post infarction syndrome. Seen most commonly after splenic, liver or other solid organ embolization.
- 24–72 hours post procedure, i.e. fever, myalgia, nausea, vominting, arthralgia, and generaly feeling ill due to release of pyrogens. Need fluid, analgesia and antiemetics. Should subside after 72 hours, if not consider infection and close monitoring. Patients should have this explained as part of consent.

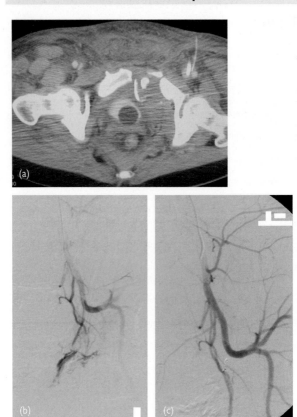

Figure 17.8 Patient involved with an RTA with pelvic fractures and dropping blood pressure. CT (a) show pelvic fracture and extravasation of contrast, confirmed at angiography (b) followed by slective embolization using a 4F glide cobra catheter (Terumo Corporation) with two 3mm x 3cm coils (Cooks UK).

Tumour ablation

This chapter will focus on the methods of tumour ablation including radiofrequency ablation, alcohol injection, and cryotherapy.

Percutaneous ethanol injection (PEI)

- The longest established technique of regional therapy for small hepatocellular carcinoma (HCC).
- It is inexpensive and easily performed under imaging guidance.
- Radiofrequency ablation (RFA) has reduced the role of PEI in the management of HCC and is now limited to treatment of particularly small tumours or as an adjunct in the management of residual disease following RFA.
- PEI can also be used in combination with transcatheter arterial chemoembolization (TACE)

Indications
- Treatment of hepatocellular carcinoma without extra hepatic disease or vascular invasion, which are not surgical candidates.
- Small and solitary lesions preferable.

Contraindications
- Deranged clotting (this should be corrected, although the risk of bleeding is smaller than that of radiofrequency ablation which requires placement of larger electrodes).
- Child – Pugh class C cirrhosis.

Note: Ascites is not an absolute contraindication, but if large in volume then consider draining first. Be sure that this does not herald Child's C disease.

Technique
- Check the platelets, clotting and correct any abnormalities.
- Review imaging and confirm the location of the tumour.
- Choose the most appropriate imaging guidance; PEI is most commonly performed under real-time ultrasound guidance.
- Conscious sedation and local anaesthesia are usually administered.
- Choose approach – transhepatic approach to the tumour is preferable to reduce the risk of painful ethanol leakage back along the needle track.
- Infiltrate with local anaesthetic to the liver capsule.
- A 20–22 gauge, end hole or multiside hole needle is used for PEI.
- For small lesions insert the needle into the distant aspect of the tumour under ultrasound guidance. Larger lesions will require multiple needle positions.
- Injection is performed in a small amounts (0.1–0 .2 ml) of absolute alcohol under continuous ultrasound monitoring. As the tumour becomes echogenic the needle is withdrawn and injection continued until the entire tumour is echogenic or the target volume is reached.
- The target volume is calculated using the formula $V = 4/3 \pi (R+0.5)$. V is the target volume and r the radius of the lesion in centimetres. This volume is as an approximate guideline as diffusion through the tumour

may be heterogeneous and in larger tumours injection will occur at more than one point.

- After completing the injection the needle is left in place for 1 to 2 minutes before withdrawing whist aspirating.
- Leakage of absolute alcohol into the peritoneal cavity is extremely painful and will require opiate analgesia to be available immediately.
- The patient is returned to the ward for bed rest with a protocol for observation of T, P, and BP. Complications include bleeding and pain.

TIPS AND TRICKS:

- Lesions near the dome of the diaphragm may be difficult to identify on ultrasound and CT guidance can then be helpful. US/CT fusion is useful if you have it.
- Residual areas of arterial contrast enhancement, due to residual tumour following incomplete thermal ablation, can be identified and targeted using ultrasound contrast agents or contrast enhanced CT.
- If multiple needles are to be used it is easier to place all needles under ultrasound control before starting the injection so that the ensuing echogenicity does not interfere with placement.
- PEI particularly useful in combination with RFA for residual or recurrent disease or lesions which are anatomically unfavourable for RFA (proximity to adjacent vessels or heat sensitive structures susceptible to collateral thermal damage).

Follow up

Contrast enhanced CT most commonly used. Early imaging allows appropriate re-treatment to be performed quickly.

Results

- As with any treatment for HCC, survival is dependent on histologic grade, Child-Pugh score, size, and number of lesions.
- In Child's A patients with a solitary tumour less than 3 cm 5-year survival rates similar to surgical resection can be achieved.
- In general terms radiofrequency ablation can achieve more predictable volumes of tumour necrosis, which are often larger, in fewer treatment episodes.

Radiofrequency ablation (RFA)

This is a minimally invasive treatment for primary and secondary liver tumours, lung tumours, renal cell carcinoma, and some soft tissue or bone metastases. RFA utilizes thermal energy to produce coagulative necrosis within the target tissue. Currently, RFA is more mature than other thermal ablative techniques (microwave, laser, cryotherapy) and produces larger treatment volumes with a low complication rate.

Indications
- Primary or secondary malignant liver tumours.
- Primary or secondary lung tumours.
- Renal cell carcinoma.
- Symptomatic bony or soft tissue metastases.

Typically, patients are unsuitable for surgical resection, although with improving RFA technology the technique is beginning to rival surgical resection in specific clinical circumstances.

Technique
- Check the platelets, Hb, clotting, and correct any abnormalities. Assess renal and liver function. Check FEV for lung RFA.
- The procedure can be performed under conscious sedation or general anaesthetic.
- Antibiotic cover is administered in the author's institution, it is not universal.
- Can be performed under real-time ultrasound, CT guidance, at laparoscopy or open laparotomy. The choice of guidance is governed by local availability, expertise and the accessibility/visibility of the lesions.
- Grounding pads are placed on the patient's thighs and connected to the RF generator. Current can then flow from the RFA electrode to the grounding pads in a similar way to diathermy.
- The RFA electrode is positioned within the target tumour and the radiofrequency energy is deposited from the RF generator.
- The duration of treatment is dependent upon different factors from the differing RFA manufacturers. Systems may be based upon a time (Tyco), impedance (Boston Scientific) or temperature (RITA).
- Electrodes are available in either straight or umbrella configurations. All the electrodes have an unshielded tip of various lengths designed to produce tissue necrosis of varying sizes.
- The geometry of the ablation zone is typically an elongated or squashed sphere (depending on the RFA system). In larger tumours it is necessary to reposition the electrodes or place several at the outset to build up overlapping spheres of ablation. The aim is to ablate the entire tumour volume with a small surrounding rim of normal tissue.
- The ablation is concluded by performing a tract ablation in which the heated electrode is withdrawn along the access tract to reduce the risk of tumour seeding and bleeding.

Patient selection

Selection criteria vary between units. Stricter criteria ensure optimal outcomes, but may exclude some patients who could benefit. Selection criteria will continue to develop as the technology of radiofrequency generators and electrodes continues to evolve.

Liver

- Most units will treat up to five lesions, <4 cm in diameter. Some will have less restrictive criteria, for size and number of lesions.
- Metastatic disease should be liver dominant with either no, or limited stable, extra hepatic disease.
- The majority of metastatic disease is colorectal carcinoma, although other tumour types are also treated.
- Patients will typically be unsuitable for surgical resection.
- Patients with hepatocellular carcinoma should have preserved liver function (Child-Pugh A&B) and not be eligible for transplantation.

Lung

- Stage I lung cancer.
- Pulmonary metastatic disease (Figure 18.1).
- 'Rule of 3's' - <3 lesions, <3 cm diameter, <3 cm from chest wall (the latter rule can be relaxed with increasing experience).

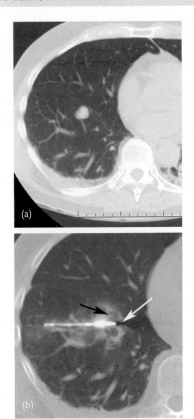

Figure 18.1 Metastatic colorectal carcinoma. 2 cm preliminary deposit (a) is treated with a multi-tined electrode (b). Artefact from the tip of the central core can be visualised (white arrow) as can the position of the tines (black arrow).

Kidney

(see 📖 Chapter 11)

- Renal cell carcinoma.
- Stage 1a disease is most suitable.
- Tumours up to 4 cm have a high rate of total ablation. Above 5 cm the complete ablation rate falls rapidly to about 25%.
- Peripheral, exophytic lesions are more easily ablated than central tumours.
- Lesions should be more than 1 cm from the ureter or renal pelvis/PUJ to minimize the incidence of collecting system or ureteric damage.

TIPS AND TRICKS:

- Scrutinize the imaging on a 3D workstation. The relationship to structures susceptible to collateral damage may be best appreciated off axis. The position of the tines of the electrodes and the relationship to tumour are best appreciated in more than one plane.
- Become familiar with post ablation imaging appearances. Detection of recurrent or residual disease in arterial enhancing lesions is relatively straightforward (Figure 18.2). For lesions which do not demonstrate avid contrast enhancement the ablation zone should encompass the entire lesion, and some surrounding normal parenchyma. This will result in an apparent increase in the size of the lesion, which should not be mistaken for disease progression (Figure 18.3). Tumour recurrence can be subtle (Figure 18.4).
- Use hydrodissection by injecting 5% dextrose to prevent collateral thermal injury adjacent structures. Useful to protect bowel and gallbladder. Remember to image during the ablation as dextrose will diffuse and the displaced structure may move back into the area at risk.
- Add non-ionic contrast to 5% dextrose (15 ml per 500 ml dextrose) to distinguish injected fluid from adjacent structures on CT.
- Interposition of an angioplasty balloon or injection of carbon dioxide can also be used as protective manoeuvres.
- Electrodes with an umbrella configuration are particularly useful for small exophytic renal tumours, which may move away from a straight needle during respiration.
- Biopsy of renal lesions is recommended. Biopsy is best performed after the initial placement of radiofrequency electrodes so that any biopsy related haemorrhage does not obscure electrode placement.
- Centrally placed renal tumours have a higher incidence of subsequent haematuria and a higher incidence of incomplete ablation.
- Administration of 25 ml of contrast at the outset of a renal RFA procedure allows visualization of the collecting system on CT. Larger volumes result in striation of static contrast in the ablation zone preventing assessment of margins on the immediate post ablation CT.
- Ureteric stent placement and pyeloperfusion (either antegrade or retrograde) with 5% dextrose can protect the renal collecting system from thermal injury during treatment of centrally located tumours.
- Expansion of the lung into the costophrenic recess with the patient prone may obscure or limit access to upper pole renal tumours. As long as the lesion lies sufficiently medially then placement of the patient with the ipsilateral side down can achieve access to the tumour and minimize ipsilateral lung inflation.
- GA is preferable when treating large or multiple lesions as times may be long and patient movement or discomfort will not limit the ablation.
- The future development of bipolar electrodes will allow continuous delivery of power between two electrodes eliminating the need for grounding pads and providing faster, larger, ablations.

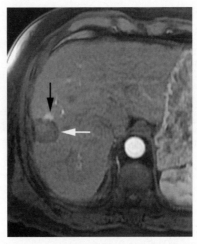

Figure 18.2 Recurrent HCC at the ablation margin. Post contrast MRI demonstrates a focal area of avid arterial enhancement (black arrow) at the anterior limit of the ablation zone (white arrow).

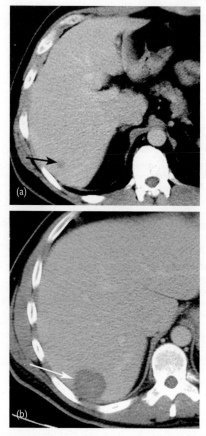

Figure 18.3 Hepatic metastases. (a) Small hepatic deposit (arrow) in this patient with three hepatic metastases. (b) Day 1 post ablation the ablation zone completely encompasses the lesion and includes a rim of surrounding normal liver (arrow). Over time the ablation zone will reduce in density and become well defined with subsequent shrinkage.

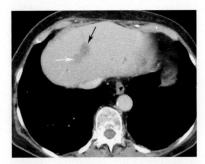

Figure 18.4 Recurrent metastatic colorectal carcinoma adjacent to ablation zone. The recurrent nodule (white arrow) is of subtly higher attenuation than the adjacent ablation zone (black arrow) and returns increased signal on STIR MRI sequences.

Follow up

- Clinical and imaging follow-up is necessary. CT/MRI is performed at 3 months, 6 months, 12 months, and annually. MRI can be particularly helpful in identifying residual or recurrent tumour in liver RFA.

Complications

Complications are uncommon.
- Abscess formation.
- Pneumothorax (28% in pulmonary RFA, but only 10% require aspiration/drainage).
- Bleeding.
- Thermal damage to the adjacent organs (gall bladder, bowel, renal collecting system/ureter).
- Biliary strictures can occur when treating perihilar lesions.
- Overall morbidity is up to 10%.
- Pulmonary RFA may have a higher mortality than other sites.

Results

- Three prospective trials of renal RFA with over 100 tumours exist and demonstrate short term effectiveness. However, no long term survival data exists for renal RFA. Imaging follow up has shown complete ablation in 90–100% of tumours less than 4 cm (Figure 18.5).
- 1- and 5-year survival rates of 78% and 27% for stage I non small cell lung cancer and rates of 87% and 57% for colorectal pulmonary metastases. Overall 30 day mortality was 3.9%.
- The outcome of RFA in the liver is critically dependent upon patient selection and factors such as the size and number of lesions and the presence or absence of extra hepatic disease as well as the prevalence of other treatments (e.g. chemotherapy) within the study population. In patients with multiple lesions 5-year survival between 18% and 30% have been reported. Patients with just a single metastasis less than 4 cm can achieve 5-year survival rates of up to 40%.

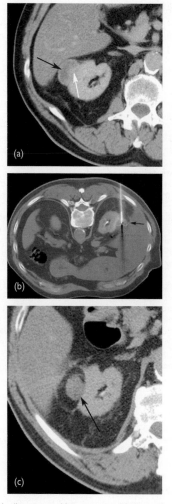

Figure 18.5 Renal cell carcinoma. (a) 3 cm tumour (black arrow), with nodular enhancement (white arrow). (b) Second ablation cycle with a multi-tined electrode (arrow). (c) 12 month follow-up demonstrating tumour shrinkage and lack of contrast enhancement (arrow).

Cryoablation

Cryoablation is currently used almost exclusively in the kidney. It utilizes cycles of freezing and thawing to produce cell death and tumour necrosis. Recent production of small calibre of cryoprobes now means percutaneous treatment is feasible.

- The cryoprobe is positioned in the tumour under imaging guidance.
- Argon gas is pumped to the tip of the cryoprobe to produce an ice ball.
- The ice ball formation causes cellular dehydration, osmotic shifts, and cell death. In addition, there is microvessel damage causing tissue ischaemia, which further contributes to tissue necrosis.
- The critical temperature, resulting in uniform necrosis lies between -20°C and -40°C. The clinical endpoint is therefore a target temperature of -40°C at the cryoprobe. The temperature at the edge of the ice ball measures zero to -10°C.
- The ice ball is monitored using CT.
- Placement of multiple cryoprobes approximately 15 mm apart allows coalescence of individual ice balls. The aim is to envelope the tumour within the ice ball.
- Two freeze-thaw cycles are administered. The freeze cycle lasts 10 mins, followed by an 8 min. thaw cycle, a further freeze cycle and a thawing cycle during which should be cryoprobes are removed when they reach 15° C.
- It is necessary to maintain the ice ball 1 cm or more from adjacent structures at risk of thermal injury.
- Generally less painful than radiofrequency ablation and therefore more suitable to conscious sedation.
- Produces a more oblong area of ablation compared with the more spherical geometry of RFA.
- A thermocouple for temperature monitoring can be placed adjacent to the zone of ablation for real time monitoring of the effect of cryoablation on adjacent structures.
- Limited but encouraging data available on follow up.

Further reading

Breen, D.J., Rutherford, E.E., Stedman, B. *et al.* (2007) Management of renal tumours by image-guided radiofrequency ablation: experience in 105 tumours. *Cardiovasc Intervent Radiol* **30**: 936–42.

Gervais, D.J., McGovern, F.J., Arellano, R.S. *et al.* (2005) Radiofrequency ablation of renal cell carcinoma: Part 1, indications, results, and role in patient management over a six-year period and ablation of 100 tumours. A.J.R. **185**: 64–71.

Gervais, D.J., McGovern, F.J., Arellano, R.S. *et al.* (2005) Radiofrequency ablation of renal cell carcinoma: Part 2, lessons learned with ablation of 100 tumours. A.J.R. **185**: 72–80.

Geshwind, J.H., Rilling, W.S. (eds) (2002) Current management of hepatocellular carcinoma. J.V.I.R. **13**(9).

Gillams, A.R., Lees, W.R. (2004) Radiofrequency ablation of colorectal liver metastases in 167 patients. *European Radiology* **14**: 2261–7.

Simon, C.J., Dupuy, D.E., DiPetrillo, T.A. *et al.* (2007) Pulmonary radiofrequency ablation: Long-term safety and efficacy in 153 patients. *Radiology* **243**: 268–75.

Siperstein, A.E., Berber, E., Ballen, N. *et al.* (2007) Survival after radiofrequency ablation of colorectal liver metastases. 10-year experience. *Annals of Surgery* **246**: 559–67.

Embolotherapy in oncology

- Useful tool in a variety of clinical situations in oncology patients.
- Can be applied to haemorrhage from ruptured hepatic tumours, a pre-operative tool or to palliate pain from symptomatic bone tumours.
- Transcatheter chemoembolization is the mainstay of treatment for a large number of patients with unresectable hepatocellular carcinoma (HCC).
- Portal vein embolization can increase the safety of extensive hepatic resection.
- Radioembolization (SIRT) is an emerging technique in the treatment of primary and secondary hepatic neoplasms.
- A sound basic grounding in the principles of embolization, a detailed knowledge of the properties and limitations of the various embolic materials, and an in-depth understanding of the relevant vascular anatomy is essential.
- It is important to observe good technique throughout, and in particular, the regular monitoring of embolization is pertinent to vessel occlusion in tumour vascular beds as flow dynamics may change during the procedure with potentially important consequences (Figure 18.6).

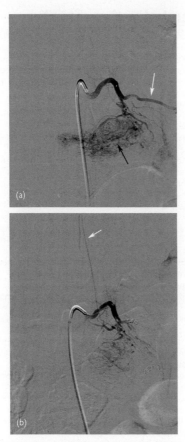

Figure 18.6 Vertebral embolization. (a) Pre-operative embolization of a vertebral body (L2) metastasis from renal cell carcinoma. The right and left second lumbar arteries have been embolized and there is further supply from the left L1 lumbar artery. Selective injection fills the distal vessel (white arrow) and the pathologic circulation (black arrow). (b) the distal artery has been embolized with microcoils to provide distal protection and divert subsequent particulate emboli to the pathologic circulation. After partial particulate embolization the interim angiogram demonstrates filling of the anterior spinal artery (white arrow), identified by the characteristic hairpin bend, not previously visible.

Chemoembolization (TACE)

TACE is predominantly used in the treatment of hepatocellular carcinoma but is also described in the management of metastatic disease.

- TACE utilizes the dual blood supply to the liver and the fact that a normal liver receives the majority of its blood from the portal vein, whereas liver tumours receive their predominant supply from the hepatic artery.
- TACE involves the intra-arterial administration of chemotherapeutic agents which are emulsified in an oily medium, followed by installation of an embolic material.
- Despite the widespread use of TACE the technique is poorly standardized and multiple regimes exist.
- TACE aims to deliver high concentrations of chemotherapeutic agent within the tumour. The addition of embolic material causes tissue ischemia, which is likely to be synergistic in achieving tumour necrosis, and the lack of arterial inflow increases the duration of contact to the chemotherapy.
- The most common chemotherapeutic agent is doxorubicin. Chemotherapeutic agents may also be used in combination and a cocktail including doxorubicin, cisplatin and mitomycin is the most widely used.
- Lipiodol accumulates preferentially within HCC and is used as a suspension medium for the chemotherapy.
- Optimal tumour response requires multiple sessions of TACE and therefore maintaining arterial patency is key to repeating the procedure.
- The selectivity of TACE remains controversial, with advocates of lobar versus segmental injection.
- TACE using drug-eluting beads (loaded with doxorubicin) has been performed in small numbers and preliminary data from the PRECISION trials is encouraging.
- Likely to create two treatment strategies depending upon tumour burden. Patients with widespread or multiple tumours will be suitable for conventional oily TACE administered to the entire lobe. Patients with more localized disease may be better suited to superselective TACE using doxorubicin-loaded beads injected selectively into the feeding vessel(s).
- Despite the worldwide acceptance of TACE, a survival advantage over embolization alone (TAE) not been proven to date.

Patient selection

- Remains controversial and it is difficult to predict accurately which patients will benefit most from the procedure.
- A variety of scoring systems exist, but none are ideal for prognostication.
- The Child-Pugh score provides a marker of underlying liver function, while the CLIP score attempts to include tumour morphology into the algorithm.

The palliative nature of the procedure should be understood by all relevant parties.

It is clear that patients with advanced liver disease, a large tumour burden, and multiple comorbidities withstand TACE less well.

In general contraindications include:

- Greater than 50% liver replacement.
- Child's C disease.
- Hepatic encephalopathy.
- Prior biliary reconstruction is a major risk factor for the development of post procedure abscesses.

Portal vein occlusion has been considered a contraindication, although there is now evidence to the contrary if embolization can be performed sufficiently selectively.

Technique

- Establish the diagnosis. This can be achieved on the basis of typical imaging features and a markedly elevated alpha fetoprotein. Less clear cases may sometimes require biopsy.
- Obtain informed consent.
- Check the platelets, clotting, liver, and renal function.
- Give antibiotics, antiemetics, and intravenous hydration.
- Conscious sedation and local anaesthesia are administered.
- Perform visceral angiography to determine the vascular supply, assess accessory or replaced hepatic arteries and patency of the portal vein. Non-hepatic branches should be identified to minimize non target embolization.
- Coil embolization of non-hepatic branches can be useful to protect the distal vascular bed in these territories.
- A catheter is advanced into the right or left hepatic artery to perform a lobar treatment and beyond for selective treatment. Whole liver chemoembolization is associated with a potential for serious impairment of hepatic function and should be avoided.
- Microcatheters are useful for selective embolization or tortuous anatomy.
- If TAE/TACE is performed for neuroendocrine hepatic metastases there can be significant peri-procedural hormonal release and prophylactic medical therapy with somatostatin analogues is required even in the absence of significant symptoms in the resting state.
- The chemotherapy agent is emulsified with lipiodol by injecting carefully between two syringes via a three-way tap. This emulsion is then administered via a correctly sited catheter. Chemoembolization with DC beads does not utilize lipiodol and the loading of the beads is performed prior to the procedure in pharmacy.
- Significant shunting to the portal vein may be encountered and will require embolization prior to administration of the chemotherapeutic mixture.
- Opiate analgesia may be required.
- Embolization is performed to reduce arterial inflow using either gel foam or particulate embolic material. The aim is to reduce inflow while maintain patency of the feeding artery.
- Patients typically remain in hospital for about 48 hours. Post embolization syndrome is common.

- Biochemistry is repeated in three weeks and a repeat chemoembolization or treatment of the contra lateral lobe can be performed after four weeks.

Results

Interpretation of the literature is difficult given the heterogeneous nature of the patient population.

- There are multiple single centre experiences of TACE but relatively few randomized controlled trials.
- Early randomized trials failed to demonstrate survival benefit for TACE but were criticized for poor trial design.
- The two most recent prospective randomized trials demonstrated a survival advantage over symptomatic management.
- Embolization has a well established role in the treatment of hepatic neuroendocrine metastases with particularly satisfactory results in the control of hormonal symptoms (control in over 90%).
- In the majority of cases embolization for neuroendocrine tumours is without the addition of chemotherapeutic. However for carcinoid tumours there is evidence to suggest TACE may be beneficial over TAE in patients with islet cell tumours.

Portal vein embolization (PVE)

- Portal vein embolization useful adjunct to major hepatic resection by inducing selective hepatic hypertrophy for patients in whom the future liver remnant is too small to allow safe resection.
- Particularly relevant to patients with cirrhosis.
- A detailed understanding of the segmental anatomy of the liver, portal vein anatomy, and the frequent anatomical variants is a pre-requisite (Figure 18.7).
- A clear understanding of the proposed resection is also essential to ensure correct embolization and accurate assessment of the future liver remnant using volumetric software applied to a CT data set.
- PVE redirects portal flow to the non embolized liver causing selective hypertrophy within the future liver remnant.
- Rates of hepatic regeneration are lower in patients with cirrhosis but despite this a useful increase in the volume of the future liver remnant can be achieved.

Indications

- Patients undergoing major hepatic resection with borderline or inadequate future liver remnant (FLR).
- The adequacy of the future liver remnant is determined by the ratio of FLR to total estimated liver volume (TELV). In patients with normal hepatic function an FLR/TELV ratio of at least 25% is recommended. In patients with significant hepatic dysfunction this increases to 40%.
- Patients with less than 18% FLR/TELV ratio are unlikely to obtain sufficient hypertrophy to achieve the required ratio to allow extensive resection.

Technique

- Transhepatic access to the portal vein is required. It is obtained using ultrasound guidance and a 5 or 6F sheath is inserted into a peripheral portal vein.
- PVE can be performed via an ipsilateral (portal access through the liver resection site) or contra lateral (portal access through the future liver remnant) approach.
- The contra lateral approach has the advantage of more direct catheterization of the right portal vein branches, but the disadvantage of possible damage to the future liver remnant. A completion portogram is more easily achieved from contralateral access.
- Catheter manipulation is more complex from an ipsilateral approach and usually requires use of reverse curve catheters.
- Embolization can usually be performed through standard 035 catheters although microcatheters are occasionally useful.
- In order to achieve maximal liver hypertrophy it is important to perform as complete an embolization as possible.
- If segment IV is to be embolized this is usually performed before right portal vein embolization (within the same procedure).
- A variety of embolic materials are described. Use of particulate material (PVA), often in conjunction with coils or glue (N-butyl-2-cyanoacrylate – NBCA)/lipiodol embolization are the most common.

- Whatever embolic agent is used embolization should include the small peripheral portal tributaries and the occluding agent should be permanent.
- NBCA/lipiodol embolization has the advantage of being achieved more quickly than particulate embolization. It is more easily performed from a contralateral approach. Use can be difficult in patients with reduced hepato-petal flow or altered hepatic flow dynamics.
- Following PVE changes in liver function tests are usually minimal and transient. 50% of patients show no change in biochemical markers. Any rise in transaminases is usually maximal on day 1-3 and has returned to baseline by day 7-10.
- Much better tolerated than hepatic arterial embolization with a low incidence of post embolization syndrome.
- Morbidity is higher amongst patients with chronic liver disease. Overall, complications occur in up to 10% with subcapsular haematoma, haemobilia, and portal vein thrombosis amongst the more common.

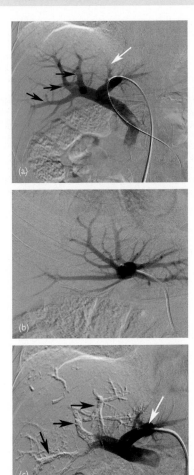

Figure 18.7 Portal vein embolization. Right portal vein embolization prior to right hepatic lobectomy. Contralateral approach from the left portal vein, (a) Portogram demonstrates right portal vein branches (black arrows) and segment IV branches arising from the left portal vein (white arrow). (b) selective left portal injection fills segment II, III and IV branches. (c) Following right portal vein embolization with glue the embolic material is visible in the right portal vein branches (black arrows), the left portal vein and branches (including segment IV) remain patent (white arrow).

Selective internal radiation therapy (SIRT)

- Emerging technique in the management of the hepatic metastatic disease and HCC which involves embolization with microspheres loaded yttrium 90(Y^{90}).
- The procedure combines internal brachytherapy with embolization.
- Y^{90} is available as either glass or resin microspheres. The resin microsphere preparation is more widely available.
- Y^{90} is a pure β emitter with a tissue penetration of approximately 2.5 mm.
- This is a complex treatment which requires a multidisciplinary team involving interventional radiology, radiation biology, nuclear medicine, and oncology.
- Meticulous angiographic technique is required to minimize complications.
- Non-invasive vascular imaging with CTA and MRA is capable of providing useful information prior to angiographic work up. However, there is no substitute for high quality digital subtraction angiography as many of the vessels are beyond the special resolution of non-invasive techniques. DSA also has the advantage of providing information related to flow characteristics unavailable with cross-sectional imaging.

Indications

- Unresectable primary or metastatic liver tumour.
- The liver involvement should represent the dominant tumour burden.
- Life expectancy greater than 3 months.

Contra indications

- Significant hepato-pulmonary shunt.
- Vascular anatomy likely to result in significant radiation dose to the gastrointestinal tract that can not be corrected by transcatheter embolization.
- Limited hepatic reserve.
- Prior radiotherapy involving the liver.
- Portal vein compromise (unless superselective SIRT can be performed).

Pre-treatment work up

- Treatment is based on disease assessment using cross-sectional imaging and hepatic vascular anatomy as demonstrated by angiography.
- Treatment is individualized to each patient.
- Preliminary imaging includes a three-phase contrast enhanced CT and/or gadolinium-enhanced MRI to assess hepatic tumour burden and distribution.
- PET-CT can be valuable in identifying occult extra hepatic disease.
- Baseline assessment of renal and liver function.
- Pretreatment hepatic arteriogram with ^{99m}Tc MAA injection to assess hepato-pulmonary shunting.

Planning angiogram and pretreatment embolization

- The initial angiographic evaluation includes superior mesenteric and coeliac angiograms, as well as selective right and left hepatic arteriograms.
- In order to prevent inadvertent deposition of microspheres within the gastrointestinal tract the hepatic artery is isolated by coil embolization of all extra hepatic branches. Identification of the small extra hepatic branches which may be encountered less commonly, or may be less important in procedures such as chemoembolization, requires extensive knowledge of hepatic vascular anatomy and its variants.
- ^{99m}Tc MAA is injected into the hepatic artery to assess shunting to the lung by performing a lung scan which should be undertaken within 1 hour of injection to prevent overestimation due to free technetium.

Y^{90} treatment

- Dosimetry is performed from pretreatment imaging and and investigations.
- Dose reduction is required in patients with limited hepato-pulmonary shunts.
- Repeat angiography is performed. Previously embolized vessels can recanalize quickly and it is important to confirm that the liver remains the sole recipient of injected microspheres. Any new vessels which have developed will require further embolization.
- Depending on anatomical considerations and institutional preference treatment can be performed in a whole liver or lobar fashion.
- Microspheres are injected into the target vessel with intermittent angiography to assess flow characteristics, which will evolve during the treatment.
- Treatment is often stopped if there is slowing of antegrade flow in order to prevent reflux and non target embolization.
- Special radiation protection measures are required to ensure the safe administration of Y^{90} and to monitor for possible spillage/contamination.
- A post procedure Bremsstrahlung scan is sometimes performed within 24 hours of treatment to evaluate the distribution of Y^{90}.

Toxicity

- Acceptable toxicity has been demonstrated in patients with metastatic colorectal carcinoma and HCC.
- Acute toxicity is typically constitutional (fever, fatigue, post embolization syndrome), gastrointestinal (nausea, vomiting, abdominal pain, and GI ulceration) or hepatic (impaired liver function).
- Late toxicity relates to radiation effects to the liver with elevated liver function tests, fibrosis and portal hypertension.

Results

- No large-scale, prospective, randomized trials exist but there is an increasing body of case-control series in patients with primary and secondary liver tumours and several small prospective randomized trials.
- SIRT has demonstrated effectiveness in salvage therapy of metastatic colorectal carcinoma.

- Phase II and phase III data have shown increased response rates and time to progression of hepatic mCRC in comparison with hepatic arterial chemotherapy or systemic 5-FU fluorouracil/leucovorin.
- A small study has demonstrated an advantage to the addition of SIRT to first line treatment with FOLFOX chemotherapy in mCRC.
- Several studies have demonstrated encouraging response rates in patients with HCC and SIRT may become an alternative to TACE.
- Small series exist documenting the treatment of metastatic breast and neuroendocrine tumours, and also cholangiocarcinoma.

Further reading

Bilbao J.I., Reiser M.F. (2008) *Liver Radioembolization with Y^{90} Microspheres*. Springer-Verlag, Berlin.

Brown D.B., Geshwind J.H., Soulen M. *et al.* (2006) Society of the interventional radiology position statement on chemoembolization of hepatic malignancies. J.V.I.R. **17**: 217–23.

Liu D.M., Salem R., Bui J.T. *et al.* (2005) Angiographic considerations in patients undergoing liver-directed therapy. J.V.I.R. **16**: 911–35.

Madoff, D.C., Gupta S., Kamran A. *et al.* (2006) Update on the management of the neuroendocrine hepatic metastases. J.V.I.R. **17**: 1225–50.

Madoff D.C., Hicks M.E., Vauthey J.-N. *et al.* (2002) Transhepatic portal vein embolization: anatomy, indications and technical considerations. *Radiographics* **22**: 1063–76.

Biopsy and drainage

Image guided biopsy

Indications
Any radiologically detected and accessible abnormality for tissue diagnosis.

Contraindications
- Abnormal coagulaopathy (INR >1.5, platelets <50000) (may give FFP if urgent).
- Uncooperative patient.
- Inaccessible lesion.

Patient preparation
- Informed consent.
- Coagulation screen/correct abnormal coagulation.
- IV access for administration of medications as and when necessary.
- Patient fasted for 2 hours before procedure.

Equipment
- Needles: the choice of needle is dependant on the specimen required by the clinicians.
  - Fine gauge needle: to obtain samples for cytology (FNAC). A 21 or 22G needle (e.g. Chiba) is used.
  - Cutting or core biopsy needle: used for larger samples for histology.
  - These are 14–18G in size with 1 cm or 2 cm variable throw.
  - These needles could be used manually (e.g. Trucut, Baxter Healthcare, USA) or with an automated device (e.g. Biopty, Bard, USA) (Figure 19.1).

Technique
Fine needle aspiration cytology (FNAC)
- Instill local anaesthesia to skin and subcutaneous tissue.
- Advance needle into the lesion under image guidance.
- Attach 20 ml syringe to needle.
- Aspirate the syringe while moving to and fro within the lesion.
- Squirt the contents onto slide and cytology smear is prepared.
- Specimens are air dried or sent in cytology containers as per local practice.

Core biopsy (automated device technique)
- Instill local anaesthesia to skin and subcutaneous tissue.
- Make 3–5 mm superficial skin incision.
- Identify the target lesion and decide on the length of the throw (1 or 2 cm).
- Advance core biopsy needle either 1 cm or 2 cm proximal to the intending target site under image guidance.
- On firing, the automated mechanism obtains the specimen.
- The needle is withdrawn and the core is expressed into formalin container for histology.

Co-axial technique
Identical to technique as above, except a 14 gauge or large needle is placed first adjacent to lesion and then a smaller longer 18 gauge or less needle is placed inside and used for the biopsy. Multiple cores can be taken without repeated needle removal.

Choice of route
Shortest route from skin to lesion avoiding vital structures.

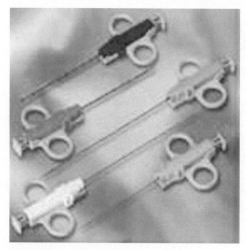

Figure 19.1 Cutting biopsy needles.

Radiological guidance
- Ultrasound (USG):
  - Appropriate probe selection to localize lesion.
  - Assess path, depth, and angle.
  - Use transducer guide if available.
  - Advance needle tip parallel to USG beam into target.
- Computed tomography (CT):
  - Perform scan of lesion in biopsy position (IV contrast to assess vascular structure).
  - Place localizing markers (e.g. paper clips on tape) at chosen level.
  - Repeat scan at the marker site.
  - Assess entry point, depth, and angle.
  - Place needle and confirm tip position on further CT.
- Fluoroscopy:
  - Lesion identified on screening (e.g. bone lesion).
  - Advance needle under biplanar screening into lesion.
  - Biopsy obtained as per standard technique.

Post procedure care

- Depends on site of biopsy, patient condition, and coagulation status.
- Chest radiograph following lung biopsy.
- Monitor vital signs, pulse, BP, oxygen saturation every 15 mins for 1st hour, every 30 minutes for the next 2 hours and hourly for 2 hrs.
- Analgesia as required.

Complications

- Liver biopsy:
  - Haemorrhage (intraperitoneal -0.7% and subcapsular up to 23%).
  - AV fistula (5.4%).
  - Infection, biliary sepsis (0.3%).
- Renal biopsy:
  - Haematuria 3–5%.
  - AV fistula.
  - Infection (0.2%).

Key points

- Multiple passes may be needed to obtain satisfactory sample.
- Avoid biopsy from necrotic centre.
- Avoid vital vascular structures and hollow viscous.

Image guided drainage

Indications
Diagnostic and/or therapeutic management of fluid collections.

Contraindications
- Coagulopathy.
- Unsafe access route.
- Unco-operative patient.

Patient preparation
- Informed consent.
- Coagulation screen.
- Other relevant blood tests, e.g. haemoglobin.
- IV access.
- Antibiotics, where indicated.
- Fasting – 2 hrs pre procedure.
- Sedation and analgesia may be required depending on patients and access.

Equipment
- Access devices: 18–21G needle depending on viscosity of the fluid, access and wire used, i.e 0.18 wire will go through 21G and 0.35" 18G. Abbocath-T (Hospira, Donegal, Ireland) very useful and safe for introducing a plastic cannula for aspiration or 0.35 (Figure 19.2) wire access prior to drainage.
- Dilators and sheaths: size depending on size of drain (e.g. 6Fr–22Fr).
- Drainage catheter: most drains are pigtail shaped and made of polyurethane material and a hydrophilic coating (Figure 19.3).
- Size of drain depends on viscosity of collection.

Type of collection	Size of drain
Clear fluid-thin pus	8–12F
Thick pus-debris	12–22F

- Fixation devices: these are often neglected and good fixation is a vital part of the procedure. In addition to internal locking mechanism (e.g. locking pigtail) most drains require external fixation to prevent dislodgement (Figure 19.4):
  - Home made (e.g. suture fixation, adhesive ostomy device).
  - Custom made devices (Molnar disc, StatLock-Venetec, USA).
- Drainage systems:
  - Closed drainage system: connecting tube, 3-way tap and drainage bag.
  - Sump drainage: draining and sump lumen to prevent cavity collapsing and blocking drain holes.

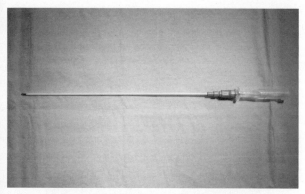

Figure 19.2 Abbocath-T. This can be used with CT or US guidance to access collections. When pus is aspirated the outer plastic cannula is advanced slightly and the inner metal needle removed. The plastic cannula will then allow delivery of a still 0.35 for drain insertion.

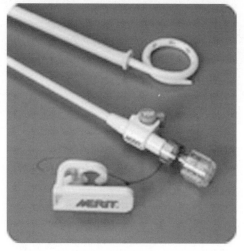

Figure 19.3 Typical locking pigtail drain. © Cook.

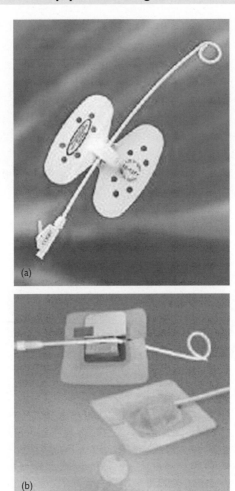

Figure 19.4 Examples of commercial fixation devices. © Cook.

Technique

Choice of route

Shortest route from skin to lesion avoiding vital structures, i.e. for pancreas and pancreatic collections several routes depending on the area or collection to be accessed may be used (Figure 19.5). For pelvic collections if no trans-abdominal route is available, a drain can be inserted via the sciatic notch (Figure 19.6).

Radiological guidance

Useful to assess:

- The site of the collection – to assess path of drainage.
- The content of collection – can influence size and number of drains.
- Choice of image guidance depends on site of collection (e.g. CT for deep abdominal and pelvic collection), preference of operator and availability of the imaging modality.
- Ultrasound(USG):
  - Appropriate probe selection to localize collection.
  - Assess path, depth, and angle.
  - Use transducer guide if available.
  - Advance needle tip parallel to USG beam into target.
- Computed tomography(CT):
  - Perform scan of region to be drained in appropriate position (IV contrast to assess vascular structure).
  - Place localizing markers (e.g. paper clips on tape) at chosen level.
  - Repeat scan at the marker site.
  - Assess entry point, depth, and angle.
  - Place needle and confirm tip position on further CT.
- Fluoroscopy and MRI guidance are used very rarely.

Drainage procedure (coaxial technique)

- Instill local anaesthesia to skin and subcutaneous tissue.
- Make 3–5 mm superficial skin incision.
- Identify the target using appropriate imaging modality.
- Advance access needle (Abbocath-T) into the intending collection site under image guidance.
- Aspirate to confirm position.
- Advance guide wire through needle to secure access.
- Withdraw needle retaining access wire.
- Use dilators to widen the track 1F–2F over the size of chosen drain.
- Advance the drain with inner stiffener over the wire into the collection.
- Detach stiffener from the drain, fix it, and advance the drain over the wire.
- Remove stiffener and wire allowing the drain form,
- Ensure free drainage to confirm position,
- Perform post procedure imaging (if required) to confirm drain placement.
- Fix drain with appropriate device and connect to drainage system.

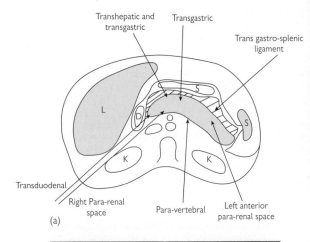

(a)

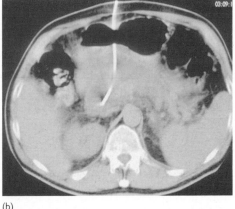

(b)

Figure 19.5 (a) Different access routes to the pancreas. (b) CT guided transgastric drainage of pancreatic pseudocyst.

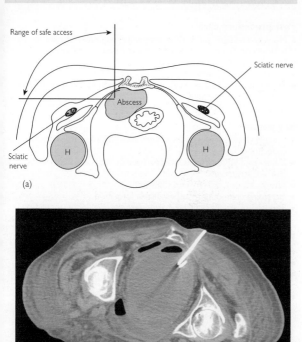

Figure 19.6 (a) Access through the sciatic notch is best in the 90 degree angle shown. This avoids the sciatic nerve shaded in grey and vessels, particularly if you stay near the sacrum/coccyx. Ideally patient is positioned semi-prone to give direct route down. (b) Sciatic route drain.

Post-procedure care

- Monitor vital signs, pulse, BP, oxygen saturation every 15 mins for 1st hour, every 30 mins for the next 2 hrs and hourly for 4 hrs.
- Continue antibiotics as required.
- Monitor drainage volume.
- Thick viscous collection may require regular (8–24 hourly) irrigation with saline and aspiration.
- Remove drain when collection is resolved and drainage stops.

Key points

- Success rate of drainage ranges from 80%–100%, lower in complex collections.
- Major complications include sepsis, haemorrhage, and injury to adjacent structures.
- Always advance drain over a stiff wire.
- Increasing drain output-suspect fistula formation.
- Reduced or absent drainage – consider reimaging in the above two situations and when there is persistent fever.

Plugged biopsies

- In patients with impaired coagulation and ascites.
- Biopsy samples with Tru-cut needle in the conventional manner.
- Outer cutting sheath left in the liver and plastic cannula inserted down the sheath.
- Gel foam/coils instilled while sheath is withdrawn.

Complex drains

TIPS:
Locules within collections may be broken up using guidewires and catheters or consider Tpa.

Transgastric drain
- Useful for draining pancreatic pseudocysts.
- Avoids pancreatico-cutaneous fistula.
- Kit identical to that of gastrostomy.
- Performed under fluoroscopy with USG or CT.
- The anterior and posterior stomach walls needs puncturing.
- Double pigtail drain is inserted across the pseudosyst and stomach lumen for internal drainage.
- Drain removed endoscopically following confirmed resolution of the collection.
- Do not drain pancreatic necrosis, as the necrotic tissue may not drain easily.

Pelvic drain
- Pelvic collections are deep and relatively inaccessible.
- CT is useful for precise localization and for image guidance to drain collection.
- If collection cannot be safely accessed from anterior approach, alternatives include transrectal, transvaginal, and transgluteal routes.
- For transgluteal route use CT guidance in prone position, traverse sciatic notch avoiding sciatic nerve and gluteal vessels.

Chest
- USG guidance to drain pleural effusion and empyema.
- Standard needle and wire technique to access the collection and to site the drain.
- Connect the drain to underwater seal drain.
- Perform CXR post drain insertion to rule out pneumothorax.

Transhepatic drainage
- Drainage of large hepatic cysts/abscess.
- Usually to drain gall bladder empyema.
- Can be performed under USG or CT guidance.
- Adequate sedation and analgesia is required, as the procedure is very painful.
- Standard co axial technique to access and drain the target.

Cystotastrostomy
- This reduces the risk of percutaneous fistula in pancreatic collections.
- For long term drainage of large symptomatic pancreatic collections in the lesser sac an alternative to surgical cystogastrostomy.
- Performed either percutaneously or endoscopically through the posterior wall of the stomach under direct vision and or endoscopic ultrasound avoiding large vessels.
- Percutaneous technique involves initial transgastric drainage as described above.
- The initial drain is exchanged over a stiff wire for a short 8F double J stent (similar to a ureteric stent).

- Distension of the stomach with air aids in forming the loop in the stomach (Figure 19.7).
- Screen AP and laterally to confirm sufficient stent in both the collection and the stomach before removing the guidewire through the pusher which maintains the drain in place. Contrast can be introduced into the collection to aid visualization during deployment.
- When the stomach loop has formed, the pusher can then be removed.

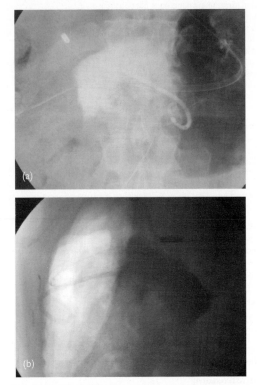

Figure 19.7 (a) AP and lateral (b) view of a cystogastromy for a chronic lesser sac pseudocyst Contrast has been instilled into the sac to aid visualization of the collection during deployment.

Pancreatic Phlegmon

Surgery may be required to drain very thick collections, particularly where there is severe pancreatic necrosis. However, where surgery is not desirable these can be drained using large drains and irrigation, although this can take some time with using large 20–24F drains.

Cholecystotomy

- High-risk and critically ill patients with acute cholecystitis – calculous/acalculous.
- Ultrasound/fluoroscopic/CT guidance.
- Transhepatic route is associated with less risk of bile leakage.
- T fastners are useful for anchoring the GB wall to the anterior abdomen.
- Transperitoneal route is preferred for stone removal through a larger tract.
- Access the gall bladder using Seldinger technique or direct trocar technique.
- Dilate the tract and place catheter over a guidewire.
- Leave on open drainage.
- Leave drain in for at least 7–10 days to allow tract maturation.
- Evaluate tract maturation before the catheter is removed by injecting contrast (Figure 19.7).
- Technical success: 98–100%.
- Complications: biliary peritonitis, bleeding, haemobilia, catheter dislodgment (5–10%).
- Death (30-day mortality 3%).

Retroperitoneal

- Retroperitoneal collections include perinephric abscess, psoas abscess, peripancreatic collections.
- CT is useful for localization and image guidance usually with patient in prone position.
- Contrast enhanced scan is useful to identify vascular structures.
- Standard coaxial technique to access the collection and to site the drain.

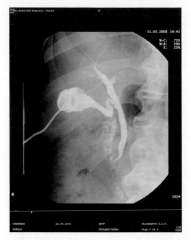

Figure 19.8 Cholangiogram following cholecystectomy confirming gallstones in the GB but free drainage in to the duodenum.

Transvenous biopsy

Indications
- Transjugular liver biopsy in patients with ascites and abnormal coagulation.
- Intravascular lesions, cavo-atrial tumours via transjugular or trans-femoral approach.

Equipment
(transjugular liver biopsy)
- Standard angiography kit.
- 5F sheath and Cobra catheter.
- Guidewires (hydrophilic and stiff wires).
- Transjugular liver biopsy set – 7Fr long sheath, angled metallic stiffener, cutting biopsy needle (Cook, UK).

Technique
- USG guided IJV puncture and introduce 5F sheath.
- Access right hepatic vein with Cobra catheter and hydrophilic wire.
- Perform venogram to confirm position.
- Exchange for stiff wire.
- Exchange 5F sheath for long 7F sheath form the biopsy set and advance into hepatic vein.
- Rotate until the directional indicator on the sheath is anterior.
- Advance cutting needle under fluoroscopy through the sheath into the liver parenchyma.
- With suspended respiration biopsy is obtained by pressing the inner stylet.
- Repeat if sample not adequate.

Key points
- Capsular perforations, intraperitoneal haemorrhage (<5%).
- Transvenous biopsies can also be performed via femoral route.

EUS guided biopsy and drainage

Indications
- Biopsy: perigastrintestinal, posterior mediastinal, aortopulmonary window, and subcarinal lymph nodes for staging.
- Biopsy of submucosal GI tumours, adrenal and pancreatic lesions.

Equipment
- Electronic linear scanning endoscopes (e.g. Pentax, Olympus).
- EUS biopsy kit either FNA or Trucut needles.

Patient preparation
- Performed as outpatient procedure.
- Fasting for 4–6 hours pre procedure.
- Standard sedation for endoscopy.

Technique
- Place transducer in a stable position in front of the targeted lesion.
- Position the lesion cranial in the image.
- Advance needle with stylet up to the inner surface of the gastrointestinal tract.
- Advanced needle into the lesion under USG.
- Reintroduce stylet to exclude obstructing tissue inside needle and remove it
- Create low pressure with 10 ml syringe and move needle to and fro.
- The low pressure is released while the needle is still in the lesion.
- Retract needle into sheath and remove entire needle assembly from the scope.
- Prepare FNA specimen slide by standard technique.

EUS guided drainage

Indications
- Drainage of pancreatic pseudo cysts.
- Drainage of pelvic collections via transrectal or transvaginal route.
- EUS guided biliary drainage, perioesophageal medistinal collection.

Equipment
- Electronic linear scanning endoscopes (e.g. Pentax, Olympus).
- Large gauge needle knife (e.g. Zimmon needle knife, Cook, USA)
- EUS FNA needle (22G) with 0.018 wire; 19G FNA needle and 0.035 wire.
- Diathermy.
- 7–10F stent and pusher catheter.

Technique
- Locate the contact zone between the gastric or duodenal wall and the cyst.
- Perform Doppler assessment for interposed vessels.
- Puncture cyst using a 19G FNA needle and aspirate for analysis.
- Perform contrast study of the cyst to confirm anatomy.
- Introduce needle knife through the working channel and puncture the cyst.
- Withdraw metal part of needle knife leaving the Teflon catheter in the cyst.
- Dilate the tract using a 6 mm or 8 mm balloon over the wire.
- Insert either a nasocystic drain or stent across the cyst wall.

Key points
- The yield of EUS-FNA is about 90–95%.
- The sensitivity and specificity of FNA is about 90% and 100%, respectively.
- Perform Doppler for interposed vessels before puncturing cyst wall.

Miscellaneous

Deflating a stuck foley catheter

- Cut the end off the foley catheter. Pass a guidewire, i.e. stiff terumo, either the floppy or stiff end, into the balloon channel and push hard. This will either release the kink or pop the balloon.
- Direct puncture with a long 22/20 gauge needle percutaneously under US guidance or CT directly onto the Foley balloon in the bladder.
- Over inflate the balloon and burst it (as long as it is not stuck in the urethra).

Pericardial tap

The depth of fluid should be >1 cm. Subcostal/subxiphisternal root is safest. Patient should be semi-erect to gravitate fluid. US guidance pass an 18 gauge needle or 14 gauge abbocatheter into the collection. Pass a guidewire, followed by a 5F pigtail catheter. May need larger catheter if it heavily blood stained.

Further reading

Kessel, D., Robertson, I. (2005) *Interventional Radiology: A survival guide* 2nd edn, Elsevier (Churchill Livingstone).

Phillips-Hughes, J. (2007) Invasive and interventional uses of endoscopic ultrasound. *Br J Radiol* **80**(949): 1–2.

Vilmann, P., Saftoiu, A. (2006) Endoscopic ultrasound-guided fine needle aspiration biopsy: Equipment and technique. *Journal of Gastroenterology and Hepatology* **21**(11): 1646–55.

Salivary and lacrimal ducts intervention

Salivary duct intervention

Common conditions
- Salivary gland obstruction due to calculi and ductal stricture are the commonest complaints affecting this organ.
- Salivary stone lithotripsy and extraction and balloon ductoplasty are carried out under imaging guidance.
- Mobile stone, or fragment, in the extra glandular part of the parotid or submandibular duct offer better results.

Contraindications
- Active infection.
- Large stone.

Kit
- 3.0 Gauge needle.
- 0.035 stiff wire and 0.018 platinum plus wire.
- 5Fr straight flush catheter.
- Lacrimal dilators.
- 2.4F stone basket.
- 2 mm balloon.

Techniques/Tips
Anaesthesia
- Standard local anaesthesia.
- IV sedation as required.

Procedure
- Standard local anaesthesia.
- Perform sialogram.
- Advance guide wire beyond stricture or stone.
- Advance balloon over the wire and dilate the stricture.
- Advance balloon beyond stone, inflate and withdraw to facilitate stone removal.
- Perform post procedure sialography.

Complications
- Infection – suspect if the pain increases 24–48 hrs after the procedure.
- Ductal rupture – might require surgical intervention.

Key points
- Basket retrieval of calculi is most effective in retrieving mobile stones in the extra glandular parotid and submandibular ducts.
- Simple, inexpensive, low-morbidity outpatient procedure.

Nasolacrimal duct intervention

Common indications
Epiphora due to lacrimal duct/sac obstruction caused by stones and stricture.

Contraindications
- Dacrocystitis.
- Post traumatic stricture (relative contraindication).

Kit
- Cannulation needle.
- Lacrimal dilators.
- Short shaft 0.14/0/18 system.
- 3 mm angioplasty balloon.
- Nasolacrimal duct stent (Cook, Europe).

Techniques/Tips
Anaesthesia
- Topical anaesthesia (e.g. 0.5% amethocaine hydrochloride).
- Infraorbital block (may occasionally be required) with 2% lidocaine.
- IV sedation as required.

Antibiotics
- Oral prophylactic ampicillin for 24 hours before the procedure
- Continue ampicillin and topical antibiotic-steroid eye drops for 7 days after the procedure.

Procedure
- Cannulate duct.
- Perform contrast study to assess the duct.
- Advance wire across stricture/stone.
- Inflate balloon to treat lesion (inflate to 30 sec).
- Flush stone fragments with saline out of nasolacrimal ducts into nose.
- Post procedure contrast study to confirm duct patency.
- Consider stenting in recurrent symptoms.
- Nasolacrimal stenting has over 95% technical success rate, up to 80% initial clinical success rate, with limited long term patency.

Complications
- Infection – suspect if the pain increases 24–48 hrs after the procedure.
- Ductal rupture – might require surgical intervention.

Key points
- Avoid damage to lacrimal canaliculi.
- Avoid repeated instrumentation of lacrimal sac to prevent scarring.
- Traumatic strictures respond poorly to balloon dilatation.
- Stenting lacrimal ducts has shown limited success.

Further reading

Brown, J.E. (2006) Interventional sialography and minimally invasive techniques in benign salivary gland obstruction. *Seminars in Ultrasound, CT, and MRI* **27**(6): 465–75.

Song, H.Y., Kang, S.G., Yoon, H.K., Sung, K.B. (1999) Nasolacrimal duct stenting. *Techniques in Vascular and Interventional Radiology* **2**(1): 32–8.

Foreign body retrieval/ repositioning: arterial, venous, soft tissue

Introduction

In the last two to three decades, the number of minimally invasive and interventional techniques involving the implantation and use of foreign objects/devices for monitoring, diagnostic and therapeutic indications – both elective and emergency (e.g. coils for embolization) has increased rapidly. For these reasons, the number of elective implant removals (e.g. retrievable IVC filters, ureteric stents) and procedure related complications with the loss or the unsuccessful/incomplete removal of implanted objects (e.g. broken catheter/wire tips, coils) has also rapidly increased.

Common types of foreign bodies

- **Vascular/Cardiac:** catheter fragments, embolization coils, guidewire fragments, vena cava filters, retained/misplaced sheaths, pacemaker/defibrillator wires, port-a-cath fragments, cardiac valve fragments, endovascular stents.
- **Non-vascular:** stents – G.I (oesophageal, colonic); bronchial; hepatobiliary, ureteric stents.

Kit

- Snares: e.g. Gooseneck snare 2–25 mm (Figure 21.1) (MediMark, Europe), En-snare (Inter-V) (Figure 21.2).
- Endovascular forceps (e.g. Cook, Europe, 3F in diameter).
- Baskets: e.g. Dormia baskets (Boston Scientific).

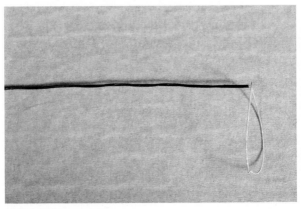

Figure 21.1 Goose neck snares.

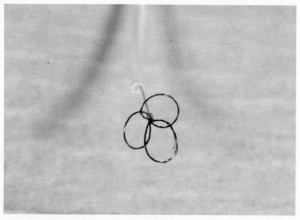

Figure 21.2 Ensnare with 3 loops at right anlges to each other.

Technique

Snares

(see Figure 21.3)

- Select snare diameter appropriate to the vessel diameter.
- Place appropriate sized sheath.
- Advance outer guiding catheter to FB.
- Advance snare/ rotate to engage FB.
- Advance guide catheter to grip FB.
- Micro snares are available for retrieval of small objects like emboliza-tion coils (Figure 21.4).
- The En-snare is a device which has three interlaced loops in one device, which makes it easier to capture foreign bodies.

Home-made snares

Home-made snares can be made with a 0.018" guidewire (Terumo) doubled back on itself through a guide catheter, forming a loop and also with a Cobra with side holes.

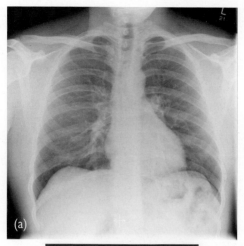

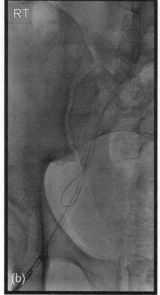

Figure 21.3 (a) Broken PICC line migrated into the right pulmonary artery.
(b) Snared and retrieved with a Ensnare through a 6F groin sheath.

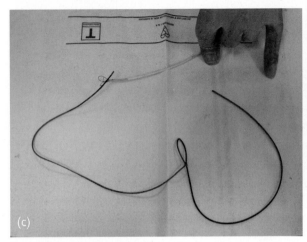

Figure 21.3c *(continued)*

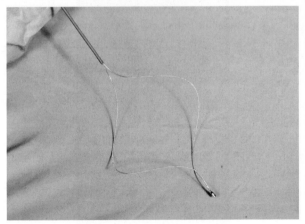

Figure 21.4 MicroElite snare.

Forceps
(see Figure 21.5)

- Small endovascular forceps (Cook, Europe) (3F in diameter).
- Have manoeuvrable tips with side-opening or end-opening jaws.
- Place forceps alongside or proximal to the object to be retrieved.
- Open the jaw to grasp the target and retrieved.
- Forceps are difficult to control under fluoroscopic guidance and may produce significant vascular injury.

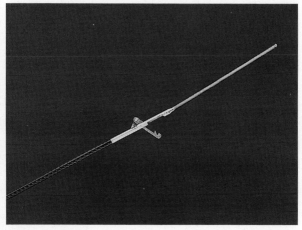

Figure 21.5 Grasper. © Cook.

Baskets
(see Figure 21.6)

- Dormia baskets (Boston Scientific) are useful to retrieve FB in the urinary or biliary systems.
- These are traumatic to vascular endothelium for use in the vascular system.

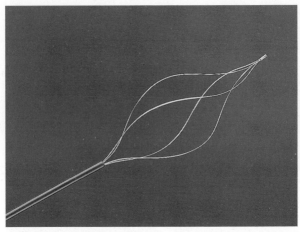

Figure 21.6 Basket. © Cook.

TIPS:

Vascular

- Access: femoral. Alternate access: cervical (mainly venous), brachial, axillary.
- Standard sheath (5–14F), dependant on the size of FB.
- A rough guide is twice the size of the FB.
- The FB can be retrieved to the mouth of the sheath, tightly snared and all removed together.
- A surgical cut-down once the FB is at the mouth of the sheath, if it is too large.
- Commonest kit: Nitinol snare (size depends on diameter of vessel), flexible grasping forceps, stone baskets.
- Foreign body grasped with kit and withdrawn into large sheath and removed.

Tips: A shaped catheter, e.g. an Sos Omni used to hook FB in difficult situations (Figure 21.7).

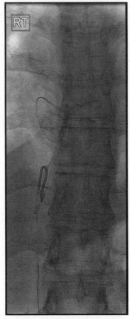

Figure 21.7 SOS omni used to hook a PICC line in the right atrium and re-orientate it down the IVC to make snaring easier.

TIPS:

Non-Vascular

Access: through natural orifice – bronchial/GI/urethral.
- To retrieve malpositioned or migrated stents and to exchange ureteric stents.
- Commonest kit: grasping forceps, snares.
- Endoscopist assistance might be useful in retrieving stents in certain difficult circumstances.

Key points
- Retrieval of FB should be attempted if it is only clinically indicated.
- Check coagulation status and correct if necessary.
- Anticipate any complications.
- Work in close cooperation with the clinical team.

Further reading

Gabelmann A., Kramer S., Gorich J. (2001) Percutaneous retrieval of lost or misplaced intravascular objects .*Am J Roentgenol.* **176**(6): 1509–13.

Wolf F., Schernthaner R.E., Dirisamer A., Schoder M., Funovics M., Lammer J. *et al.* (2007) Endovascular management of lost or misplaced intravascular objects: experiences of 12 years. *Cardiovasc Intervent Radiol.*

Musculoskeletal intervention

Introduction

There is a growing role for image guided percutaneous injection to joints and soft tissues. While many of these treatments are long established in the clinical setting, there are clear advantages to the use of imaging guidance. Safe and effective therapeutic doses can be delivered predictably to the target joint or soft tissue area. Focal areas affected by disease processes can be targeted specifically and the imaging itself has a diagnostic and follow-up role.

Almost all of the interventions can be achieved with access to a C-arm fluoroscopy unit or ultrasound machine. These techniques should not pose equipment or significant cost issues for radiology departments. These services can provide an invaluable asset for local musculoskeletal specialist and primary care providers.

Joint and bursal injections

General principles

Sterile technique

Sterility essential. Aseptic technique must be used as far as possible. The skin should be thoroughly cleaned with an antiseptic preparation which should be allowed to dry. A sterile drape with a small aperture is then applied to the skin. A sterile field is required on a trolley. If ultrasound is used, sterile probe cover and sterile gel should be applied.

Consent

Informed consent must be obtained prior to any intervention (see 📖 Chapter 1). The patient should be warned of possible post-procedure ache and pain and be given a contact to get in touch with if there are specific problems.

Efficacy

Although there is strong anecdotal data, there is little in the way of controlled evidence to support corticosteroid injections into joints and soft tissues. However, many clinical guidelines from clinical societies support their use. Meta-analyses do support short but not long term benefit varying from weeks to 2–3 months. Evidence on tendon injections and techniques such as autologous blood injection is developing but is mainly in the form of uncontrolled case series.

Contraindications/cautions
- Active soft tissue or joint infection (except for diagnostic aspiration).
- Coagulopathy including therapeutic anticoagulation (relative depending on the procedure).
- Allergy to agents used.

Complications

The adminstration of local and corticosteroids is generally safe and well tolerated with appropriate patient selection and sterile techniques.
- Symptom flare/synovitis: may occur in up to 5%. Is usually short-lived and may be a crystal effect of corticosteroid.

- Allergy: low risk if no previous history.
- Systemic steroid effects: may cause facial flushing. Blood glucose control may be impaired in diabetics.
- Tendon weakening/rupture: rare but many authors advise avoiding multiple injections around tendons within a short time period (3 months).
- Avascular necrosis: reported but causal effect controversial.
- Septic arthritis: rare if sterile technique is used. Estimated risk is 1 in 15,000.

Aftercare

It is good practice to observe the patient for a short time after the procedure to exclude reaction to the medication used or delayed vasovagal episodes. For many of these procedures this can be relatively informal, e.g, the patient may be asked to sit outside the room with a drink for 20 minutes prior to leaving.

We recommend that a responsible adult comes with patients to drive or escort them home safely.

For diagnostic injections, it is a good idea to provide the patient with a pain diary. This is usually based on a VAS scoring scale from 1 to 10. The completed diary can then go in the notes as a record of response. This is an important record in patients who have multiple interventions in order to plan future/further management.

Hip joint

Indications
- Diagnostic/therapeutic in arthropathy.
- Diagnostic for septic arthritis, often in paediatric irritable hip scenario.
- Diagnostic for hip prostheses loosening or infection.
- As part of MR arthrogram.

Equipment
- Small sterile pack and antiseptic solution.
- 10 ml and 5 ml syringe.
- 23G hypodermic needle for skin and 22G spinal needle for injection.
- Local anaesthetic (short acting for skin, long acting for injectate if required). Steroid solution for injectate if required. Dilute gadolinium if required for MR arthrogram.

Complications
- Femoral nerve block from LA is not uncommon and is transient.
- Post procedure aching may occur and is transient.

Fluoroscopic guidance (adult patient)
- Position the patient supine on the x-ray table.
- Mark a spot on the skin anteriorly at the mid-point of the intertrochanteric line.
- Subcutaneous LA to skin (Figure 22.1).
- Direct a 22G spinal needle obliquely along the axis of the femoral neck until bone is encountered. You should aim to contact the femoral neck about half way along its length.
- Inject contrast via a connecting tube under screening. If in the joint contrast should flow away from the needle tip and spread around the joint (Figure 22.1).
- If contrast pools at the needle tip, you are likely to be positioned within the ilio-psoas bursa. Withdraw the needle tip and reposition.
- Inject local anaesthetic (diagnostic), LA and long acting steroid preparation (diagnostic/ therapeutic).

Ultrasound Guidance (infant/child)
- Apply EMLA® cream to skin before procedure.
- Under direct US control anterior oblique approach to fluid collection with a 22G needle.
- Aspirate fluid for microbiology.

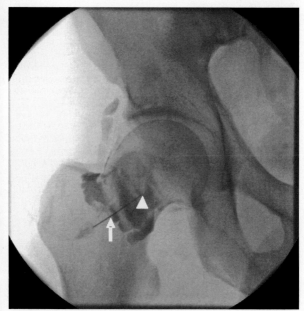

Figure 22.1 Right hip injection. The white arrow marks the site for needle skin puncture. The needle is obliquely directed along the femoral neck to contact bone at the position indicated by the white arrowhead. The joint distends with contrast.

Hip joint (prosthetic)

Fluoroscopic guidance (adult patient):

- Same technique as above – you will not see the metal needle against the prosthesis, however.
- Aim to hit metal half way up the femoral stem.
- Aspirate to obtain microbiology samples in suspected prosthetic infection.
- For suspected loosening, take control films and then inject contrast. Digital subtraction is useful when available to assess contrast leak into the bone-cement interface.
- Aspirate fluid for microbiology.

> **TIPS:**
> - If it is not possible to aspirate fluid the joint can be irrigated with a small flush of sterile normal saline.
> - A second needle inserted to the joint can be aspirated as the first needle is flushed to try and irrigate injectate around the joint.

Bursal injections around the hip

Equipment

As for hip joint injection – see above.

Psoas bursa injection

- Ultrasound control – document the presence of bursal fluid.
- Place patient supine – mark the femoral vessels on the skin.
- Anterior approach. Under direct sonographic control – advance a small gauge spinal needle deep to the iliopsoas tendon.
- Inject anaesthetic/steroid.

Trochanteric bursa injection

- Ultrasound control – document the presence of bursal fluid and the integrity of the gluteus medius and minimus tendons.
- Place patient supine – mark the injection site on the skin.
- Lateral approach. Under direct sonographic control – advance a small gauge spinal needle deep to the gluteus tendons and into any bursla distendsion.
- Inject anaesthetic/steroid.
- This technique may be combined with tendon injection for tendonosis (dry needling and autologous blood injections).

Knee joint injection

Indications

- Diagnostic/therapeutic in arthropathy.
- Diagnostic for septic arthritis.
- Diagnostic for prostheses loosening or infection.
- As part of MR arthrogram.

Equipment

As for hip joint injection – see above.

Technique

Fluoroscopic guidance (anterior approach):
- Supine position.
- Anterior paramidline approach lateral to quads tendon.
- Contrast injection to confirm position.

Fluoroscopic guidance (lateral approach):
- Lateral oblique position.
- Lateral approach aiming for back of patella lateral aspect.
- Contrast injection to confirm position.

Foot and ankle injections

Indications
Complex anatomy and motion at the mid and hind foot can make clinical determination of the source of a patient's pain difficult. Diagnostic injection may have an important role in determining pain generators.
Radiographs should be examined first – in cases of severe OA and large osteophytes, it may be worth considering a CT guided approach.
- Diagnostic/therapeutic in arthropathy.
- Long acting local anaesthetic (diagnostic) and steroid anti-inflammatory (therapeutic) as required.

Equipment
As for hip joint injection – see above.

Ankle injection
Technique
Fluoroscopic guidance
- Anterior approach. AP tube position initially. Position patient with the knee slightly flexed and the sole of the foot flat to the table.
- Mark the tibialis anterior (TA) tendon, the extensor hallucis longus (EHL) tendon, and the dorsalis pedis artery on the skin before starting. Puncture site should be medial to the artery. Puncture between the TA and EHL tendons will avoid the neurovascular bundle.
- After initial puncture, roll the patient's ankle and foot to the lateral position.
- As you advance follow the needle with a lateral tube position and guide into the joint space.
- Plantar flexion may help to open up the joint space.
- Contrast injection to confirm position (Figure 22.2).
- Document any communication with the subtalar joint (10%) or FHL tendon sheath (20%).
- 5 mls can usually be injected to the ankle joint.

Alternative technique
Ultrasound control; anterior approach with direct sonographic guidance.

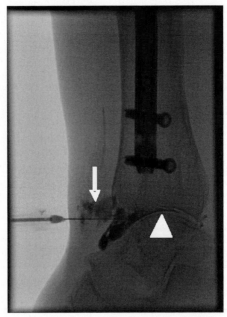

Figure 22.2 Right ankle injection. Lateral view – a 22G needle has been advanced under screening control. Initial injection is extraarticular (white arrow). Following repositioning the intra-articular space is filled with contrast (white arrowhead).

Talonavicular joint injection

The talonavicular joint often communicates with the anterior and middle subtalar joints. Therefore talonavicular injection is the preferred route of access to inject the middle subtalar joint which is difficult to access percutaneously.

Technique

Fluoroscopic guidance

- Dorsal approach. AP tube position initially.
- Slight elevation of the forefoot with padding may improve visualization of the joint.
- Mark the tibialis anterior tendon and the dorsalis pedis artery on the skin before starting.
- Direct your needle towards the joint space.
- As you advance follow the needle with a lateral tube position and guide into the joint space.
- Contrast injection to confirm position.
- 1 ml is usually the capacity of the talonavicular joint and other small foot articulations.

Alternative technique

Ultrasound control; anterior approach with direct sonographic guidance.

Posterior subtalar joint injection

Technique

Posteromedial

- Position patient in the lateral decubitus position, lateral side of the foot down.
- Position tube so that posterior aspect of PSTJ project tangentially.
- Initial puncture 1 cm posteroinferior to the pulsation of the posterior tibial artery.
- Advance needle under lateral screening to the posterior lip of the subtalar joint.
- Contrast injection to confirm position.
- Document any communication with the ankle joint.

Anterolateral

- Position patient in the lateral decubitus position, medial side of foot down.
- Position tube so that anterior end of PSTJ is parallel to the beam.
- Initial puncture.
- Advance needle under lateral screening to the posterior lip of the subtalar joint.
- Contrast injection to confirm position.
- Document any communication with the ankle joint.

CT Guided

(see Saifuddin (2005) *Clinical Radiology* **60**(2): 191–195)

- Useful technique especially in severe OA where there may be lipping osteophytes.
- Position foot in scanner to obtain coronal view of the subtalar articulation.
- Direct a needle under CT control into the joint.

- Contrast injection to confirm position – repeat scanogram is useful here to document any communication with the ankle joint.

> **TIPS:**
>
> If there is severe joint space narrowing and/or large osteophytes, CT control is generally an easier mode of access as the accessible joint space can be instantly appreciated.

Midfoot joint injection

The naviculocuneiform joint is continuous with the intercuneiform joint and the lateral cuneocuboid joint – these joints can be considered together.

The plane of the joint is oblique to AP imaging so tube angulation is required for access. A dorsal approach with oblique tube tilt is optimal for the medial joints here. Elevation of the forefoot on a pad is often helpful to improve visualization of the joint.

Forefoot joint injection

Metatarsophalangeal joints

The MTP joint space visible with an AP tube is not accessible with a vertical needle approach. The needle should be inserted 5 mm proximal to the joint and directed distally to enter the joint.

Shoulder injections

Glenohumeral joint injection

Indications
- Diagnostic/therapeutic in arthropathy and adhesive capsulitis.
- Diagnostic for septic arthritis.
- Diagnostic for prosthetic loosening or infection.
- As part of MR arthrogram.

Equipment
As for hip joint injection – see above.

Fluoroscopic control, anterior approach:
- Patient supine, AP tube.
- Externally rotate the arm, a sand bag may be used to hold in gentle external rotation.
- Mark the skin over the GHJ at the junction of upper 1/3 and lower 2/3 of the visible joint space.
- Anaesthetize the skin and subcutaneous tissues.
- Advance a 22G spinal needle into the joint.
- Inject contrast to confirm position (Figure 22.3a and b).

Fluoroscopic control, posterior approach:
This approach has been advocated in MR arthrography for anterior instability, to avoid contaminating the anterior soft tissue with gadolinium.
- The patient is positioned prone with a pad to raise the side to be injected.

- Fluoroscopy is used to ensure that the glenohumeral joint is seen tangentially.
- The inferomedial quadrant of the humeral head is targeted.
- A 22G spinal needle is advanced vertically under fluoroscopic guidance to the humeral head.
- Inject contrast to confirm position.

Ultrasound control posterior approach

- Prone position, side to be injected raised.
- Visualize the infraspinatus in longtitudinal profile. The GHJ is seen deep to the tendon.
- Pass a 22G spinal needle towards the joint until it meets the posterior aspect of the humeral head.

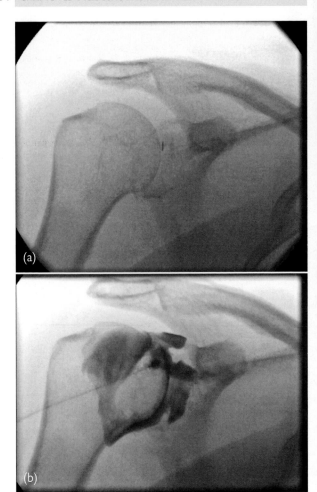

Figure 22.3 Right shoulder injection. (a) demonstrates AP view with the joint space well profiled. The site for needle puncture is marked. (b) demonstrates intra-articular spread of contrast.

Glenohumeral hydrodilation

The technique is as described for adhesive capsulitis. (see Watson L., Bialocerkowski A., Dalziel R., Balster S., Burke F., Finch C. (2007) Hydrodilatation (distension arthrography): a long-term clinical outcome series. *Br J Sports Med* **41**: 167–73).

The techniques above are used to access the joint. Subsequently, the capsule is distended with a dilute solution of steroid/anaesthetic and a subsequent saline injection until there is full distension of the subscapularis bursa, rupture down LHB tendon sheath, or pain terminates the injection.

Combined with the appropriate physiotherapy, significant benefit has been demonstrated in range of motion and pain at up to 2 years.

Acromioclavicular joint injection

Ultrasound guided

- Direct superior approach. Visualize the ACJ with the probe.
- Direct a 23G needle into the visable joint space.

Shoulder bursal and tendon injection

Indications

Diagnostic/therapeutic in impingement or tenosynovitis.

Equipment

As for hip joint injection – see above.

Subacromial bursal injection

Ultrasound guided

- Obtain a view of the supraspinatus tendon in longtitudinal profile.
- Anaesthetize the skin at the lateral aspect of the probe.
- Direct a 4 cm 21G/23G needle parallel to the superior aspect of the tendon.
- With needle resting above and parallel to supraspinatus inject a small volume of local anaesthetic. If the needle is correctly positioned fluid will flow away from the needle and distend the subacromial space.

Long head of biceps sheath injection

Ultrasound guided

- Obtain a short axis view of the LHB tendon within the sulcus.
- Direct a 4 cm 23G needle down to the groove, aiming to pass just lateral or medial to the LHB tendon itself.
- Inject local anaesthetic – if needle correctly positioned fluid will flow away and distend the tendon sheath. Injection into the tendon itself must be avoided as it can cause rupture or split.

Elbow injections

Indications
- Diagnostic/therapeutic in arthropathy.
- As part of MR arthrogram.

Equipment
As for hip joint injection – see above.

Elbow joint
Fluoroscopy guided
- Patient seated beside X-ray table.
- Elbow flexed with lateral/radial side upwards.
- Profile the radio-capetellar joint with the beam.
- Direct a 23G needle directly down to the joint space.
- Inject contrast to confirm intra-articular position.

Common extensor origin (CEO) injection (for tennis elbow)
Ultrasound guidance
- Visualize the CEO in longtitudinal aspect.
- Under direct sonographic control direct a 23G needle adjacent to the tendon.
- Treatments include steroid/anaesthetic injection around the CEO, dry needling of the tendon substance, and autologous blood injection – you should be guided by local clinicians' preference and the emerging evidence base in this area.

Wrist injection

Radiocarpal joint
Indications
- Diagnostic/therapeutic in arthropathy.
- As part of MR arthrogram.

Equipment
As for hip joint injection – see above.

Fluoroscopic guidance
- Patient seated beside table, wrist placed dorsal surface up.
- Visualize and mark the radiocarpal joint. Puncture point will be 3–4 mm distal to the visible joint space. Anaesthetize the skin locally.
- Turn wrist lateral. Advance 23 or 25G needle into joint.
- Confirm intra-articular position with contrast.

Spinal injections

General considerations

Percutaneous interventions are used in pain control and diagnosis of many spinal disorders. Specialist equipment and kit is usually not necessary.

However, with any prodecure involving the spine and meninges there are potential complications and as with any intervention, books are no substitute for hands-on teaching. Therefore, appropriate training and supervision should be sought from an experienced operator prior to embarking on these techniques.

These techniques have a variable evidence base. Their use does provide short term pain relief and they are valuable tools in conjunction with a back pain rehabilitation and physical therapy programme.

Lumbar facet joint injection

CT or fluoroscopic approach in common usage

- The facet joints are paired synovial articulations of the superior and inferior facets of adjacent vertebrae. The joint capsule is thickest posteroinferiorly where there is a synovial recess. The joints are richly innervated (from the medial branch of the spinal nerve at the level of the facet and the level above).
- Facet joint pain may manifest as low back or buttock ache, typically exacerbated by spinal extension.
- CT and MR degeneration is frequently seen but is non-specific – SPECT studies may have a role in identifying which joints to target.
- Traditionally the diagnosis is made by documenting response to a diagnostic injection.

Indications
- Diagnostic/therapeutic in suspected facet joint pain syndrome/arthropathy.

Equipment
- Small sterile pack and antiseptic.
- 23/21G hypodermic needles for skin, 22G spinal needle.
- Short and long acting local anesthetic and corticosteroid.

Risks/complications
- Septic arthritis and epidural abscess (risk less than 1 in 1,000 with good technique and sterile precaution).
- Epidural haematoma – low risk.

Efficacy
Proponents claim response of 28–54% at 3 months. However, evidence base is controversial. Injections are felt to be useful diagnostically and as part of a pain management and rehabilitation programme.

CT facet injection
Direct approach to joint under CT control.

Fluoroscopic approach

Two techniques are described:

Direct posterior (Figure 22.4)

- Position patient prone with a bolster or pillow under the abdomen to reduce the lumbar lordosis. This has the effect of distending the inferior joint recess.
- Mark the skin at the 1–2 o'clock position for the left pedicles and the 10–11 o'clock position for the right pedicles.
- Advance with a straight spinal needle under screening control until bone is encountered.
- Contrast injection is useful to document intra-articular position and any communication with the other levels.

Oblique posterior:

- Tube or patient angled to profile the facet joint directly.
- Mark the skin over the inferior joint margin.
- Advance with a straight spinal needle under screening control until bone is encountered.
- Contrast injection is useful to document intra-articular position and any communication with the other levels.

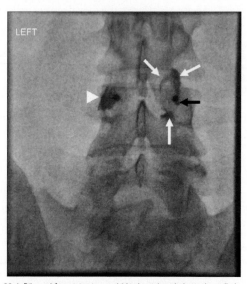

Figure 22.4 Bilateral facet injections at L3/4. the right sided spinal needle has been inserted at the 11 o'clock position on the right L4 pedicle (black arrow). Contrast outlines the facet joint on the right (white arrows). On the left contrast is pooling around the facet joint (white arrowhead) but repositioning is required to access the joint space.

Lumbar nerve root injection

Indications
Diagnostic/therapeutic.

Equipment
- Small sterile pack and antiseptic.
- 23/21G hypodermic needles for skin, 22G spinal needle.
- Short and long acting local anesthetic and corticosteroid.

Efficiacy
Short term relief of lower limb radicular pain is achieved in 60–70% and there is sustained benefit in a minority. The evidence is variable in quality and is contradictory but several studies suggest that up to 50% of appropriately selected patients may avoid surgical decompression with use of nerve root blocks.

Complications
- Temporary numbness.
- Nerve root damage and weakness.
- Spinal cord infarction (from presumed intravascular injection).

Some authors recommend use of non-particulate water soluble steroid to reduce risk.

The root should be targeted in the lateral foramen within the 'safe triangle'. The triangle is composed of a roof made up by the pedicle, a tangential base corresponding to the exiting nerve root, and the lateral border of the vertebral body (Figure 22.5). This area lessens the risk of inadvertent vascular injection.

Consideration should also be given to use of contrast to documenting that the needle tip is not intravascular.

Cervical root injections are a relatively high risk procedure and will not be covered in this discussion.

CT control
- Patient in prone position.
- Direct approach to nerve root obliquely under CT control.
- Position needle just short of the nerve root within the lateral foramen (Figure 22.6).
- Inject steroid (water soluble preparation) and LA.

Fluoroscopic control
(see Figure 22.5)
- Position patient prone with a bolster or pillow under the abdomen to reduce the lumbar lordosis.

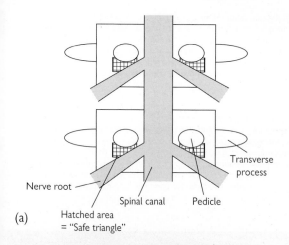

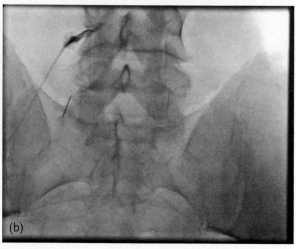

Figure 22.5 (a) The root should be targeted in the lateral foramen within the 'safe triangle'. The triangle is composed of a roof made up by the pedicle, a tangential base corresponding to the exiting nerve root, and the lateral border of the vertebral body (trianglular shaded area in schematic diagram). (b) Nerve root injection at left L4 and L5 roots. The upper spinal needle has been advanced to rest adjacent to the left L4 root. Contrast outlines the root and excludes intravascular position. The lower spinal needle is positioned at the starting point to access the L5 root – 1 cm inferior and lateral to the L5 pedicle (with thanks to Dr. D Wilson).

Find the pedicle on AP fluoro and mark it on the skin.

- Move 0.5 cm inferior and 0.5 cm lateral. Place a 9 cm 22G needle directly vertical. At about 4 cms (thin patients) to 7 cms (larger patients) turn the C arm lateral and make sure the needle tip is at the level of apex of the foramen just below the pedicle.
- If you hit osteophytes move further down and out by the same amount. Adjust forward or backward to position above the root.
- Return to AP and inject contrast agent which should track along the fascial planes obliquely along the root. Vertical contrast streaking means too deep or too shallow. Do not disconnect the extension tube but follow the contrast with the drugs whist screening to ensure the needle is not moved into a vessel or root sheath.
- Advantages are that 10 cm is not long enough to hit anything important anteriorly and the vertical approach means that you cannot hit the dura. It is also much faster and easier than an oblique approach and arguably is safer. The contrast agent injection confirms that the foraminal region will be bathed in drugs and is a vital safety check.

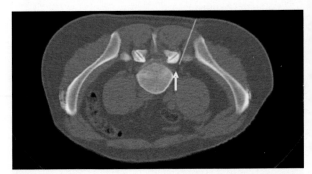

Figure 22.6 CT Nerve root injection. A 22G spinal needle has been directed obliquely to a position adjacent to the right L5 nerve root within the lateral foramen (arrow).

Lumbar provocative discography

Indications

Provocative discography is a controversial technique and there is a lack of consensus on its role in lower back pain. Advocates of the procedure utilize it to provoke pain at disc levels prior to spinal fusion operative procedures. The procedure should therefore be reserved for patients with chronic lower back pain, who are willing to contemplate surgical fusion and should be performed only at the request of the spinal surgeon in charge of the case.

Complications
- Flare of low back pain.
- Nerve root irritation.
- Post-procedure infective discitis. Some centres advocate the use of prophylactic antibiotic cover but there is no evidence base for this and antibiotic cover is not in universal use.
- A dual needle technique (co-axial) and rigorous aseptic technique should be used, however, to avoid this potentially disastrous complication.

Equipment
- Small sterile pack and antiseptic.
- 23/21G hypodermic needles for skin, coaxial spinal needle system with inner 25G 12 cm and outer 20G 9 cm needles.
- Short and long acting local anesthetic and corticosteroid.

Technique
- Fluoroscopic control.
- Local anaesthetic and/or conscious sedation may be used.
- Consent the patient for pain and infection.
- Target the levels indicated by the surgical team. A 'control' level should be included to try and document an asymptomatic disc.
- If there is lateralizing sciatica the opposite side should be used for access. The patient is positioned with this side raised by 45 degrees.
- The x-ray tube is obliqued to profile the disc space with the endplates parallel. The skin is marked at the targeted levels, cleaned and anaesthetized.
- Coaxial needle puncture with outer 19G 9 cm and inner 25G 12–15 cm spinal needles. The inner needle should puncture the annulus which is felt as a 'give' by the operator.
- A 2 ml syringe containing contrast is injected to confirm nuclear position. Pitfalls include annular injection where the periphery but not the centre of the disc fills – the needle should be withdrawn and repositioned.
- Many authors advocate manometry to measure disc injection pressures. The volume injected should be recorded and the patient's pain response carefully monitored and recorded.
- I like to inject a small amount (0.5 ml) of long acting local anaesthetic at the end of the procedure to attempt pain relief.
- The report should document the levels injected, the volume (and pressure if measured) of injectate, the patients' pre and post injection level

of pain (VAS score), and whether the pain provoked was of similar quality and location to their usual pain.
• Interpretation should be in conjunction with a spinal surgeon, ideally through an MDT process.

Percutaneous vertebral augmentation (vertebroplasty and kyphoplasty)

Vertebral augmentation is a useful tool in treating painful vertebral collapse secondary to osteoporosis or malignancy. This is a technique that must be learned hands on at the many courses available and in conjunction with an experienced operator. In the UK, the British Society of Skeletal Radiologists (www.bssr.org) is supportive in putting radiologists in touch with appropriate training.

Indications

Pain from vertebral fractures. Restoration of vertebral height is not predicable and not a worthwhile indication. In patients with multiple fracture levels marrow oedema signal (on STIR imaging) may be a useful indicator of recent or non-healed levels.

Equipment
• Large sterile pack and antiseptic.
• 23/21G hypodermic needles for skin.
• Prepacked vertebroplasty needle and delivery systems available from several manufacturers.
• Short and long acting local anaesthetic.

Contraindications

Disruption of the posterior vertebral wall (relative), coagulopathy, allergy.
• High quality C-arm (biplane is an advantage) fluoroscopy is required. Pre-packed kit containing cement, needles, and delivery systems are available from several manufacturers. Kyphoplasty is a variation on vertebroplasty where balloon dilation under high pressure creates a cavity within the affected vertebra prior to cement injection.
• Sedation and intravenous analgesia or general anaesthetic may be utilized. Under fluoroscopic control the vertebra to be treated is accessed unilaterally or bilaterally via a pedicular or parapedicular approach. A small volume (2–4 mls lumbar vertbra, 1–2 mls thoracic vertebra) of radioopaque polymethylmetacrylate (PMMA) is injected carefully under constant fluoroscopy.

Complications
• Cement leak into the canal is a rare but potentially devastating occurance.
• Chemical embolization to the lungs is also rare but may be fatal.
• Nerve root irritation occurs at a frequency of 1–2% approximately and early pain and tenderness at the site of injection is common.

Radiofrequency ablation in the musculoskeletal system

Indications
- Facet joint denervation.
- Treatment of osteoid osteoma, osteoblastoma.
- May have a role in managing painful bony metastases.

Treatment of osteoid osteoma, osteoblastoma
- CT guidance is utilized to locate the nidus of the lesion and subsequently place a thin (1 mm) RF probe into the nidus.
- A co-axial drill system is useful to penetrate the bone. 4–5 minutes if thermal treatment is sufficient.
- Reported cure rates are 90–95%. Larger lesions (e.g. osteoblastoma) may require several treatments and probe positions.

Facet joint denervation (medial branch rhizotomy)
- In patients with facet mediated pain who typically will have had temporary response to previous facet joint injections or nerve blocks.
- RF treatment to the medial branch at the level of the painful facet and the level above. The RF probe is positioned medially on the superior aspect of the transverse process.
- Low frequency testing is utilized to ensure the radicular nerves are not stimulated (this is a spinal procedure that must be learned hands-on with appropriate experience and support initially).

RF in managing painful bony metastases
There is a growing evidence base supportive of a role for RF abalation and cementoplasty in the palliation of painful bony tumours. The exact indications and role are, however evolving in this field.

Bone and soft tissue biopsy

- Any lesion that could represent a primary sarcoma should only be biopsied under the direction of a specialist unit paying strict attention to musculoskeletal compartmental anatomy.
- Tumour seeding in the biopsy track is well recognized and the biopsy track excised along with the lesion at the time of definitive surgery.
- 19% of patients with musculoskeletal tumours required a more complex resection or more radical treatment due to inappropriate biopsy technique. 5–8% of patients required an unnecessary amputation due to poorly planned biopsy.

In bone and soft tissue tumours, it is good practice to review the approach with all the relevant imaging with the orthopaedic surgeon involved. In possible sarcomas the above applies. In probable metastatic lesions careful review of anatomy should also apply. Preferably a single compartment only should be breached and care taken to avoid important neural, vascular and functional anatomy. Spring loaded cutting needles are useful for soft tissue lesions or bony lesions with significant extra-osseous components. Lesions confined to bone may be approached with cutting bone biopsy systems or drill bone biopsy systems.

Further reading

Fritz, J., Niemeyer, T. Clasen, S., Wiskirchen, J., Tepe, G., Kastler, B., Nägele, T., König, C.W., Claussen, C.D., Pereira, P.L. (2007) Management of chronic low back pain: rationales, principles, and targets of imaging-guided spinal injections. *RadioGraphics* **27**: 1751–71.

Liu P.T., Valadez S.D., Chivers F.S., Roberts C.C., Beauchamp C.P. (2007) Anatomically based guidelines for core needle biopsy of bone tumors: implications for limb sparing surgery. *Radiographics* **27**: 189–205.

Mankin H.J., Mankin C.J., Simon M.A. (1996) The hazards of biopsy revisited. Members of the Musculoskeletal Tumor Society. *J Bone Joint Surg Am* **87**(5): 656–63.

Mathis, J.M (ed.) (2004) *Image Guided Spine Interventions*. Springer-Verlag, New York.

Peterson J.J., Fenton D.S., Czervionke L.F. (2007) *Image-Guided Musculoskeletal Intervention* Saunders, Philadephia.

Silbergleit, R., Mehta, B.A., Sanders, W.P., Talati, S.J. (2001) Imaging-guided injection techniques with fluoroscopy and CT for spinal pain management. *RadioGraphics* **21**: 927–39.

Interventions in the chest

Percutaneous trans-thoracic needle biopsy

(see 📖 Chapter 19)

Indications for percutaneous trans-thoracic needle biopsy
These include diagnosis of
- Solitary pulmonary nodule not amenable to bronchoscopic biopsy.
- Pulmonary mass not amenable to bronchoscopic biopsy.
- Multiple pulmonary nodules of unknown aetiology.
- Persistent infiltrates of unknown aetiology.
- Pleural/peripheral lesions.

Contraindications
- Coagulopathy.
- Respiratory failure.
- Abnormal lung function.
- Pulmonary hypertension.

Technique CT/fluorscopy/US
- Non-invasive diagnostic imaging (computed topographic, fluoroscopic or ultrasound (the latter for pleural/peripheral lesions)), to determine the location of the lesion and planning of a suitable approach.
- Intravenous access is obtained. The patient is positioned in an optimum position to gain access to the lesion/area of lung of interest. The skin is disinfected with iodine or chlorhexidine in alcohol, then the skin, inter-costal muscles and pleura anaesthetised with 1% lidocaine. A skin nick is made with a number 11 scalpel blade.
- Under image guidance the needle (either an 18G cutting needle, e.g. Temno (Cardinal Health) or for FNA a 25G needle) is advanced into the lesion and samples taken. Compression is applied to the access site (Figures 23.1–23.2).
- A chest radiograph is performed to exclude pneumothorax/haemo-thorax.
- The patient is observed for up to 4 hrs with monitoring.

Monitoring
During and after the procedure, blood pressure, pulse, ECG, and arterial oxygen saturation monitoring is carried out.

Complications
(reported incidences for CT-guided biopsies in parenthesis)
- Pneumothorax (8–64%)
- Haemorrhage (usually minor) (2–10%)

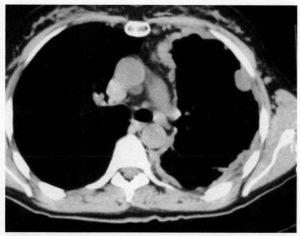

Figure 23.1 Peripherally based nodule amenable to ultrasound or CT-guided biopsy (Image courtesy of Dr. T. Meagher, Consultant Radiologist, Stoke Mandeville Hospital).

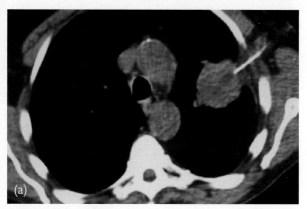

Figure 23.2a A cutting needle biopsy of left sided lung mass under CT guidance (Image courtesy of Dr. T. Meagher, Consultant Radiologist, Stoke Mandeville Hospital).

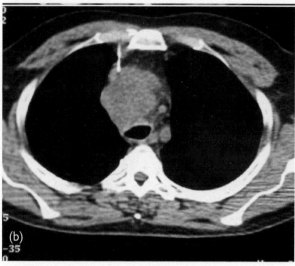

Figure 23.2b B FNA of mediastinal mass (Image courtesy of Dr. T. Meagher, Consultant Radiologist Stoke Mandeville Hospital).

Bronchial artery embolization

50% of patients with massive haemoptysis (300–600 ml of blood per day) die without treatment. Under essential anatomy.

Arises from:
- Bronchial circulation   (90%)
- Pulmonary circulation   (5%)
- Other sources (e.g. intercostal artery, axillary, and subclavian artery branches and internal mammary artery)   (5%)

Essential anatomy
- 70% arise between superior end plate T5 and inferior end plate T6.
- 45% single bronchial artery usually right one side and two the other.
- Single bilateral bronchial arteries in 30%.
- 15% sub aortic arch origin even thyrocervical trunk, internal mammary and inferior phrenic. Latter may also give separate supply as well as cos-tocervical trunk, and left gastric.
- Consistent right intercostobronchial trunk seen in 80% arising postero-laterally, others arise antero-laterally. (see Figure 18.6b).
- **Beware that the anterior spinal artery often arises from the 5th intercostal and if visualized avoid catheterization. If coming off a bleeding vessel then ensure embolization catheter is well distal and not reflux during embolization.**

Indications

Massive haemoptysis (aetiology includes malignancy, bronchiectasis, pulmonary hypertension, tuberculosis, mycetoma, and lung abscess).

Technique
- Correct any coagulopathy.
- The normal lung may require protection with selective intubation by an anaesthetist and unstable patients may require anaesthetic support.
- The cause and site of bleeding are localized using plain chest x-ray, computed tomography (with computed tomographic angiography), and fibre-optic bronchoscopy.
- Angiography alone used for both diagnosis and treatment in the acutely bleeding patient.
- Common femoral artery is punctured (usually right side) and a 5F sheath inserted.
- The bronchial artery anatomy is delineated by performing a descending thoracic aortogram (40 ml of low osmolar contrast medium at 20 ml/sec via a 4F pigtail catheter). This usually detects the abnormal bronchial artery (Figure 23.3).
- The abnormal bronchial artery is catheterized (e.g. with a Cobra catheter (Cordis, Johnson & Johnson Medical Ltd)) catheter and hydrophilic guidewire (Terumo, Terumo UK Ltd). A microcatheter is employed for selective embolization, allowing the catheter tip to be positioned in the bronchial circulation beyond any spinal cord arterial branches, thus preventing spinal cord infarction).

- Manual injection bronchial angiography is performed to confirm the abnormal bronchial artery; suggested by vessel hypertrophy, tortuosity, hypervascularity, and contrast extravasation (Figure 23.4).
- The abnormal bronchial artery is embolized using polyvinyl alcohol particles (150–250 microns for smaller vessels and mild shunting, 350–500 microns for larger vessels), absorbable gelatine sponge or coils. Avoid latter as may need to come back another time.
- If the source of bleeding is not a bronchial artery the pulmonary artery and/or other source vessels must be interrogated.

Monitoring

The degree of sedation and/or anaesthesia required will dictate the level of monitoring and should include blood pressure, pulse, ECG, and arterial oxygen saturation.

- 75–90% immediate clinical success.
- 20% reccurence at 6 months and 50% long term.

Complications
(reported incidences in parenthesis)

- Spinal cord ischaemia	(1–6.5%)
- Chest pain (usually transient)	(24–90%)
- Subintimal dissection	(1–6%)
- Dysphagia (from oesophageal arterial branch embolization)	(0.7–18%)
- Pulmonary infarction	(rare)
- Other non-targeted organ embolization (e.g. colon)	(rare)

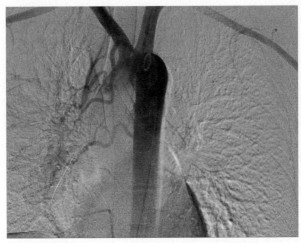

Figure 23.3 Aortogram showing abnormal subarch and decending thoracic aortic bronchial arteries.

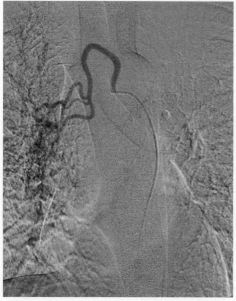

Figure 23.4 Selective right bronchial artery angiogram showing abnormal hypertrophied vessel.

Bronchial stenting

Bronchial stents are mostly placed for palliation, usually for airways obstruction. The procedure is usually performed simultaneously by respiratory physicians and interventional radiologists.

The stent is made of either silicone (e.g. Dumon bronchial stent, Bryan Corp., Woburn, MA), which requires rigid bronchoscopy for placement and is removable, or metal (e.g. Wallstent, Schneider, Inc., Minneapolis, MN) which can be inserted via a flexible bronchoscope and is permanent.

Indications
- Obstruction by malignant tumours.
- Benign strictures.
- Bronchial stenosis (post lung transplant or surgical resection and anastomosis).
- Extrinsic compression by tumour.
- Tracheomalacia.
- Airway fistulae (usually to gastrointestinal tract).
- Kyphoscoliosis causing airways compression.

Contraindications
- Non-viable lung distal to obstruction.
- Contraindications to bronchoscopy.

Technique
Covered stents are used for fistulae and bare stents for stenosis/obstruction.
- The bronchial anatomy is assessed with helical computed tomography using multi-planar reformats.
- The bronchial diameter either side of the stenosis/obstruction and the length of the stricture are measured (the respective contralateral bronchus measurements may be a useful guide).
- Bronchoscopy will allow assessment of the pliability of the stenosis and its location and length.
- The stent is then positioned under bronchoscopic and fluoroscopic guidance.
- The desired distal point is marked with a cutaneous radio-opaque marker. A guidewire (e.g. 0.035 flexible tipped) will aid stent passage in a very tight stenosis.
- If the bronchial obstruction is very tight, pre-stent placement negotiation with a guidewire and balloon dilatation may be required.
- The stent is then deployed across the stenosis from the pre-marked position to the proximal patent airway.

Monitoring
Bronchial stenting can be carried out under local anaesthesia and sedation or general anaesthesia. Monitoring will depend on degree of anaesthesia and should include blood pressure, pulse, ECG, and arterial oxygen saturation monitoring.

Complications

- Haemoptysis.
- Airways obstruction.
- Stent migration (more common in benign disease).
- Granuloma formation.
- Pneumothorax.
- Pain.
- Mucous plugging.
- Erosion through bronchial wall.

Pleural drains

(see 📖 Chapter 19)

Indications

- Pleural effusion (parapneumonic, malignant or postoperative thoracic surgery) (Figure 23.5).
- Empyema.
- Traumatic haemothorax.

Contraindications

Coagulopathy.

Technique

Simple pleural effusions can be drained using an 8–10F pigtail catheter. Empyemas require 12–16F catheters. Some interventionalists advocate larger bore drains for empyemas.

- Plain chest x-ray determines the presence of pleural fluid. Computed tomography may aid in diagnosis of an empyema, showing enhancing pleural layers and/or loculations.
- Prophylactic antibiotics are given in traumatic haemothorax.
- The patient is positioned either sat up leaning over an adjacent table, supine at 45 degrees with arm behind head or in the lateral decubitus position.
- Ultrasound confirms fluid, the presence of septations, loculations, and is used to pre-mark a safe approach at the site of the greatest depth of the collection.
- The skin is cleaned with iodine or chlorhexidine in alcohol.

Under ultrasound guidance:

- Just above a rib, local anaesthetic (1% lidocaine) is infiltrated into the skin, intercostals muscles and pleural surface. The skin is incised with an 11 scalpel blade.
- A sheathed needle (e.g. Abocath (Hospira, Belgium)) is inserted until its tip has entered the collection and effusion/pus/blood can be aspirated, and the metal stylet is removed.
- A stiff guidewire (e.g. Amplatz extra stiff 80 cm, Cook Medical, Ireland) is passed through the sheath, the latter removed, and the tract dilated over the guidewire in stepwise fashion to the desired size.
- The chest drain (e.g. pigtail catheter) is inserted into the collection over the wire and fixed by an adhesive dressing or sutured to the skin, and subsequently connected to an underwater seal.
- The size of residual pleural fluid can be monitored by chest x-ray and the catheter removed when the drainage is <10 ml per day and the patient has clinically improved.

Complications
(reported incidences in parenthesis)

- Pneumothorax   (2%)
- Haemorrhage   (1%)
- Surgical emphysema   (3%)

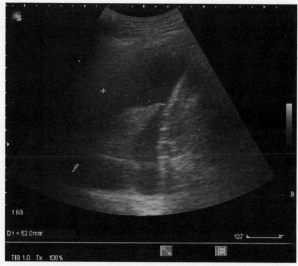

Figure 23.5 Ultrasound of right pleural effusion with measured depth. The liver is clearly seen beneath the diaphragm as is a tongue of echogenic collapsed lung.

Index

The index entries appear in letter-by-letter alphabetical order.